Borderline Personality Disorder Demystified

Effective Psychology Techniques to Combat BPD. A Borderline Personality Disorder Survival Guide

By Victor Nelson

The following Book is reproduced below to provide information that is as accurate and reliable as possible. Regardless, purchasing this Book can be seen as consent to the fact that both the Publisher and the author of this book are in no way experts on the topics discussed within and that any recommendations or suggestions made herein are for entertainment purposes only.

Professionals should be consulted as needed before undertaking any of the actions endorsed herein. This declaration is deemed fair and valid by both the American Bar Association and the Committee of Publishers Association and is legally binding throughout the United States. Furthermore, the transmission, duplication, or reproduction of any of the following work, including specific information, will be considered illegal, irrespective of whether it is done electronically or in print. This extends to creating a secondary or tertiary copy of the work or a recorded copy and is only allowed with the express written consent from the Publisher. All additional rights reserved. The information in the following pages is broadly considered a truthful and accurate account of facts. As such, any inattention, use, or misuse of the information in question by the reader will render any resulting actions solely under their purview. There are no scenarios in which the Publisher or the original author of this work can be in any fashion deemed liable for any hardship or damages that may occur them after undertaking the information described herein.

Additionally, the information in the following pages is intended only for informational purposes and should thus be thought of as universal. As befitting its nature, it is presented without assurance regarding its prolonged validity or interim quality. Trademarks mentioned are done without written consent and cannot be considered an endorsement from the trademark holder.

Table of Contents

Chapter 1

Introduction to Borderline Personality Disorder

Individuals with borderline personality disorder (BPD) battle against their feelings, actions, and sense of self, just as against their relationships with others. Since they are in such incredible pain, they frequently resort to adapting techniques that appear to work at the time but that aggravate their disorders (for example, suicide endeavors or medication use).

In reality, individuals with BPD most of the time lurch through life as though they're driving a 350-horse vehicle without any brakes.

They spontaneously act upon their thoughts without thoroughly considering things cautiously. Thus, inwardly, individuals with BPD resemble exploited people, incredibly delicate to even the scarcest trace of a feeling but so terrified of their emotions that they try to do everything without exception to stay away from them. BPD has gotten a blast of interest recently, both from analysts and well-known media. Analysts analyze what causes BPD, when and how individuals recover from BPD, the mind zones engaged with BPD, and the medications that help individuals live satisfying and fulfilling lives. You may be asking yourself, "For what reason is BPD such an interesting disorder now?"A better question would be, "Why did it take so much time for it to become a topic of interest?" After all, people with BPD experience extraordinary agony.

They battle with unwavering strength in their relationships with others, sentiments of void, loneliness, and edginess, and a confounded feeling of their identity and where they are going throughout everyday life. Up to 10 percent of individuals with BPD commit suicide, a rate more than multiple times that of healthy people.

However, despite these data, numerous individuals with BPD don't get the help they need. BPD likewise impacts the lives of relatives, companions, and parental figures. On the slight off chance that a physicist was to compose an elixir that would spread sickness, concern, and misfortune among friends and family, this mixture would presumably look a lot like BPD. It is terrible and alarming when somebody you love discusses or endeavors suicide. Attempting to assist somebody with BPD resembles being dropped into an arena full of lions and warriors that try to kill you. The intense feelings of individuals with BPD can be energizing and serious. But, on the other hand, individuals with BPD can be sensational and appealing, and they are frequently very mindful and comprehensive.

The emotional power of an individual with BPD can sear and singe connections. Furthermore, individuals with BPD frequently become gulped by melancholy or misery, leaving the parental figure or relatives unsure about what to do. Numerous individuals with BPD and their friends and family don't comprehend the troubles they battle with consistently or where to turn for help. Even though there is a sprinkling of data accessible on the web, the Internet can be a befuddling and misleading place for somebody who is suffering, with deception and sites offering dangerous advice prowling everywhere. For instance, those that promote self-damage and eating disorders. So, where can somebody with BPD turn to get valuable information? Two sources that contain a ton of information are treatment manuals and research papers.

It is helpful for individuals battling BPD to have forward-thinking, precise, and open information on their disorders and where to go to find support. Hence, we wrote the following chapters to give individuals with BPD a simple-to-follow guide to help them through the labyrinth of their disorders. The next chapters will be handy if any of the following sentences are true for you.

- You have been determined to have BPD and need to get familiar with the issue;
- You feel that you may have BPD and need to make sense of what to do;
- You hurt yourself, experience unrest, and need to learn supportive adapting skills;
- You are getting help or taking drugs and need to get familiar with BPD, its causes, and the things you can do to support yourself;
- You care for or treat somebody with BPD, and you need a conceivable wellspring of data that lets you know precisely what BPD is and what to do about it.

Chapter 2

What is Borderline Personality Disorder?

We have dedicated this part to give you a detailed, effectively reasonable picture of BPD. So on the slight chance that you believe that you or somebody near you may have BPD, it is helpful to know precisely what this implies.

Before reading this chapter, it is significant for you to realize that you can't determine yourself to have BPD. Even though you may find out about a portion of the side effects of BPD and believe "That is me!" you should see an expert (an analyst, a specialist, or another person who analyzes mental issues) make sense of whether you have BPD or not. We hope you don't from the bottom of our hearts.

Attempting to determine for yourself to have a mental disorder is like deciding for yourself to have cancer or coronary illness. You need an expert to do it since you doubtlessly don't have the devices, abilities, or perspective to reach a sound and rational conclusion.

Also, if you made an inappropriate finding, you probably won't get the correct sort of help. For example, we have met with a few people who thought they had BPD yet ended up having some other disorder, similar to sorrow, bipolar confusion, or post-traumatic stress disorder.

Similarly, as the prescribed medicines for cancer are not the same as those for diabetes , each mental or behavioral disorder requires specific treatment. Consequently, you'll have to ensure your conclusion is precise, and the best way to do this is to see an expert. So, utilize this section to realize what BPD is about but not diagnose the pathology.

Mental disorders, Personality disorders and BPD

A personality disorder is essentially a way of identifying with the world that doesn't work well with the actual circumstances. These disorders cause incredible pain and may make it challenging seeing someone or completing simple tasks in everyday life (for example, getting to work or keeping your job). There is a wide range of personality disorders, including avoidant, fanatical impulsive, needy, schizoid, schizophrenia, narcissistic, and, obviously, borderline personality disorder. Having a personality disorder implies having many mental issues that have been with you for quite a while.

For the most part, you must be a grown-up adult to be determined to have a personality disorder. In any case, individuals determined to have a personality disorder as grown-ups will regularly say that they have battled with these disorders for whatever length of time that they can recall. Accordingly, we know that numerous individuals have had these disorders since they were youngsters.

Having a personality disorder doesn't imply that you have an imperfect personality, have a poor character, or are mean or unlikable. Essentially, the popular supposition is that individuals with personality disorders have some part of their being that creates these issues for themselves and others. However, we don't agree with this, for a couple of reasons.

To begin with, the term personality disorder is hazardous because it's frequently utilized reciprocally with phrases like "personality imperfection," "disorder individual," and "troublesome personality," and, as we said previously, this use isn't precise.

Second, this term recommends that the disorder is within you and that on the slight off chance that you could fix yourself, everything would be fine. We can't help contradicting this perspective as well. There is a great deal of proof that the environment (for example, stress, injury, misuse, and other factors) assumes a solid job in numerous mental disorders, including personality disorders.

Furthermore, putting the disorder within you can make shameful and critical responses concerning others.

At long last, the term personality disorder likewise recommends that, if you have a personality disorder, you have consistently had it (its piece of your personality, some portion of what makes you the individual you are), and you generally will have it. As you'll find in the coming chapters, there is proof that BPD can be cured. Along these lines, having BPD doesn't imply that you have an imperfect personality or that you will consistently battle with the disorders you are having at this moment.

It just implies that you have a way of reasoning, feeling, and carrying on your life that might be blocking your capacity to have a good quality of life, prop your connections up, or reach your goals.
The problem with this though is that mental disorder doesn't appear to work similarly as illnesses do. In the first place, you can't "get" a mental disorder like you can get pneumonia. Secondly, dissimilar to diseases, mental clutters have not been connected to any physical breakdown that may cause them. Third, a considerable portion of the side effects of the explicit disorder are found in numerous different disorders, so the line between them is foggy. Interestingly, it is evident to doctors when an individual has diabetes versus BPD.

There is also the supposition that certain acts, feelings, or thoughts demonstrate the presence of a hidden disorder. That is a significant jump to make. Researchers can't glimpse inside somebody's body or brain and locate a primary condition, as they do when they find a carcinogenic tumor. Furthermore, the sickness model, similar to the term personality disorder, puts the disorder for the most part within you. As we depict in the following chapters, if you have BPD, a significant number of the disorders you battle with are identified with disturbances in the environment instead of conditions within you. Besides, the progressions that you may need to make to be more joyful may include changing nature or changing how you act, think, or feel. Consequently, we believe that what you do, think, and feel are considerably more significant than whether you have confusion or not.

History of BPD

The broadly held view was that there were two vast classifications of mental disorders or illness. One category, called despondency, included patients who knew about the actual world but had behavior disorders, such as sadness or nervousness.

The other classification, called psychosis, included patients who had abnormal musings and encounters that were not present in the other patients. These people were often determined to have schizophrenia. Finally, patients who didn't have disorders sufficiently genuine to be marked as crazy, but were too disturbed even to consider being called masochists, were placed into the borderline classification.

Therapists utilized the term "fringe" for patients who made some hard memories seeing both the great and terrible characteristics in individuals simultaneously, who drove insecure and noisy lives, and who were regularly genuinely in trouble. A considerable part of these perspectives about BPD came straightforwardly from perceptions of a set number of patients and did not depend on analytical research. Since those early days, specialists have led various examinations. Discoveries from these examinations have distinguished numerous significant characteristics that make up what we presently call borderline personality disorder, including challenges overseeing feelings, indiscreet conduct, and bad relationships.

Individuals with BPD are never again thought to verge on psychosis and anxiety. Science is helping us keep the thoughts regarding BPD that appear to be valid and dispose of the old ideas regarding BPD that don't seem to be exact.

Symptoms of BPD

BPD is a turmoil of insecurity and disorders with feelings. Individuals with BPD are insecure in their feelings, reasoning, connections, personality, and conduct. Individuals with BPD have rough relationships and are regularly scared of being left alone. Inwardly, individuals with BPD feel like they are on an exciting ride, with their feelings going here and there suddenly.

Likewise, they may experience difficulty with anger management. Individuals with BPD act imprudently when they are under stress, and they now and then endeavor suicide and take part in self-hurt. Frequently, individuals with BPD experience difficulty making sense of their identity, and they experience difficulty thinking plainly and staying grounded when they are worried.

In the following few pages, we will take a look at the different symptoms of BPD.

Feeling strange

This alludes to insecure feelings and trouble overseeing feelings. A few specialists have said that feeling dysregulation is the most significant disorder for individuals with BPD. In reality, a few people accept that most of the diseases that individuals with BPD battle with are brought about by feeling dysregulation. Temperamental feelings, mindsets, and trouble controlling resentment are the main manifestations of BPD that fall under this classification.

Emotions and moods

Individuals with BPD regularly respond to things that probably won't influence others so firmly. For example, on the slight off chance that you have BPD, you may be handily furious about something that an individual's state or do, or you may find that you get worried more effectively than others. Only a little bare or opposing look may be sufficient to toss you into an angry spiral. Since individuals with BPD respond genuinely to such a large number of things, they regularly find that their feelings are all over the place. They may feel glad one moment and immediately afterward miserable or angry.

Intense anger and difficulties in anger management

Individuals with BPD might be effectively aggravated or infuriated by things that probably won't agitate others.

They may not be able to control themselves when they blow up—tossing things, hollering at individuals, or feeling so devoured by rage that they don't have a clue what to do. Even though outrage is one measure for BPD, we have seen, in working with individuals who have BPD, that the feelings of shame, pity, and blame are regularly a lot stronger and harder to adapt to. A few people with BPD appear to invest more energy being angry with themselves than with others.

Relational issues

Relational issues implies experiencing difficulty when associating with others. However, it doesn't mean that you are an awful or unlikable individual. Indeed, individuals with BPD are regularly very enchanting, fascinating, and delicate.

Precarious and intense relationships

Individuals with BPD regularly have "rough" connections that are riotous and crazy. Their dynamic force makes it difficult for them to manage relationships. On the slight chance that you have BPD, you may find that occasionally things go exceptionally well in your connections, and on different occasions, everything appears to self-destruct. You might be cheerful, in adoration, and thrilled one minute, and the following minute you may feel angry and have sad thoughts about your connections.

The essential thought is that connections, similar to feelings, appear to be exciting, and they rush from excellent to downright awful. If you have BPD, your relationships may include numerous contentions, battles, and even physical or psychological mistreatment.

Behavioral issues

Conduct dysregulation implies that your conduct is wild, and possibly hurtful or unsafe, and negatively affects your life. Individuals with BPD regularly battle with this disorder in two essential manners: a dangerous conduct and self-hurt.

Identity issues

With self and personality dysregulation, an individual doesn't have a good or stable feeling of who the individual in question is and can likewise feel void a significant part of the time.

Subjective dysregulation

With emotional dysregulation, an individual encounters negative reasoning and separation from self or reality when the individual is worried. It is critical to note here that these disorders are not generally there and happen predominantly when individuals with BPD are under a great deal of pressure or are genuinely disturbed.

Stress related issues

If you are battleing with this disorder, it doesn't imply that you are silly, schizophrenic, or insane. Instead, it means that when you are worried, you begin to turn out to be particularly suspicious or stressed over how others feel about you. You may start to accept that individuals are attempting to be mean to you, exploit you, or mischief you here and there.

You may likewise believe that individuals are taking a gander at you and thinking negative or critical things about you (for example, "He's fat," "She's bad looking," "I don't care for her"). These encounters will, in general, happen when you are under pressure or are feeling vexed, yet they don't frequently occur when things are going quickly. The other part of psychological dysregulation is separation. Separation is the experience of being looked at, scattered, in a foggy mental state, not mindful of your environment, or feeling as though you are not inside your body.

Feeling of separation of the self

A few people portray this feeling as though drifting to the roof and looking down on their bodies and the individuals around them. At the point when present in BPD, separation happens under pressure. Separation can be an approach to get away from trouble. For instance, if your manager fires you and you feel apprehensive, restless, and angry, you may look at it intellectually for a brief period to escape from your disorders or your misery. The problem with separating is that it doesn't unravel anything. You may do things when you are separating that are hazardous (for example, suicide endeavors) or that you don't recollect a while later (for instance, dangerous single-night rendezvous).

How do you know if you have BPD?
As we talked about at the beginning of this book, the ideal approach to determine if you have BPD is to meet with an expert who can accurately analyze. A few distinct sorts of psychological well-being experts make analyses, including specialists and clinicians. Therapists are clinical specialists with specific preparation in prescription-based and mental medicines.

Therapists and analysts are often able to do an intensive evaluation and make a conclusion. We advise you that you look for an expert with preparing and involvement in personality disorder and that you get a careful evaluation. Since BPD includes a long-standing example of identifying with the world (and is something that numerous individuals have battled with for the duration of their lives), the way toward diagnosing BPD may take some time. Even though it tends to be difficult to be tolerant when you genuinely need to discover what's up with you, a precise determination is significant. It might require a few visits and a great deal of talking. Likewise, it is substantial that the expert you work with knows how to recognize BPD from different scatters that may look like BPD, such as bipolarism or depression.

Chapter 3

Borderline Personality Disorder: the Truths and the Myths

Analysts, clinicians, and other experts have constantly agreed that having data is fundamental to the recovery process, paying little heed to what disorders you battle with. However, it is beneficial for clinical and mental illnesses to have exact data regarding the confusion's causes, manifestations, and movement.

Moreover, on the slight chance you are battling BPD or different disorders, simply realizing that you have these disorders is a decent beginning stage. Notwithstanding, having increasingly detailed data can give you a more precise feeling of what is new with your body, brain, connections, and life when all is said and done. With this information comes a superior thought of how to address the disorders you might be having.

Right now, knowing the realities about a disorder might be one of the most significant initial phases in recouping from that clutter. Also, as you will see all through this book, we currently know a great deal about what causes BPD and what's in store on the slight off chance that you experience the ill effects of this disorder.

Tragically, however, exact data isn't in every case promptly accessible. Rather, falsehood flourishes, and it tends to be exceptionally hard to sift through the reality from the fiction and reality from the myths. This can make the path to recovery considerably more troublesome.

So it's insufficient to have recent data—it must be precise data. Also, lamentably, it appears that regardless of all the new data we are finding out about this disorder, relentless fantasies about BPD keep on driving individuals adrift and add to the shame related to this disorder.

 Albeit numerous psychological, mental disorders have a social shame connected to them, the disgrace related to BPD is particularly solid. Backing gatherings and purchaser associations like the National Alliance on Mental Illness (NAMI) have worked vigorously over the previous decade to diminish the shame appended to extreme psychological   sickness.

Subsequently, we currently observe less pessimistic depictions of individuals with these psychological disorders in the media, just as we see less falsehood spread on the web. Nonetheless, the shame related to BPD appears to endure right up to the present time. For what reason would society deride individuals with BPD more than individuals with a different disorder? Even though we don't know without a doubt, there are a couple of potential reasons.

In the first place, as of not long ago, the reasons for BPD were ineffectively comprehended, and, lamentably, at times, individuals respond most adversely to disorders they can't understand. Second, as we referenced prior, vast numbers of the side effects of BPD hit a nerve for individuals in our general public. Third, a portion of the behaviors that accompany BPD might be crazy and hard to comprehend.

For instance, self-mischief and suicide endeavors may startle and confound others, challenging to identify with. When individuals don't comprehend conduct, particularly when that conduct alarms them, it is simpler to pass judgment on the individual who is participating in that conduct than it is to put forth an attempt to comprehend that individual.

Likewise, our general public, for the most part, esteems to be quiet, relaxed, gathered, and in charge—something that individuals with BPD frequently battle with. But, for sure, because individuals with BPD have exceptionally compelling feelings and regularly express these feelings in outrageous or sensational manners, individuals who are worth being in charge of emotions may pass judgment on individuals with BPD, and they may even create negative convictions about individuals with BPD.

The profound feelings and stunning practices seen in BPD may frame the premise of social disgrace about BPD. At last, another wellspring of shame might be TV and movies. The media appear to be attracted to

BPD. Individuals with BPD can be emotional, energizing, and appealing, and the media can use the power of their encounters to gather more views.

So it is most likely not a surprise that TV and filmmakers are keen on delineating such solid, extreme, and emotional personalities. The problem here is that in trying to get excellent appraisals for the emotional impact, the media will generally portray uneven and oversimplified portrayals of BPD that are typically negative.

Antagonistic, mistaken, and hardhearted depictions of individuals with BPD are seen routinely. Even though it is likely not done with a bad attitude, these depictions add to the shame connected to BPD and make it harder for people in general to truly comprehend this disorder.

Borderline personality disorder and myths
We believe it is essential to clear up the generally normal and irrational fantasies about BPD.
Subsequently, what follows is a list of the seven irrational myths on BPD.

- Myth 1: People with BPD are manipulative and attention-seeking
- Myth 2: People with BPD are violent individuals, at high risk for harming others
- Myth 3: BPD is a life sentence
- Myth 4: BPD is not curable
- Myth 5: BPD is caused by bad parents
- Myth 6: People with BPD are crazy and irrational
- Myth 7: BPD is only found in women

Chapter 4

What Causes Borderline Personality Disorder?

Remember that no one is 100 percent sure about what causes BPD. In any case, discoveries from numerous investigations in the most recent years have proposed that BPD results from a blend of hereditary qualities, science, personality characteristics, and upsetting encounters.

One significant inquiry that you may have is whether you can acquire BPD from your parents. One way specialists have attempted to respond to this inquiry is by leading investigations with twins. Fundamentally, scientists have taken a few arrangements of twins and hoped to see whether indistinguishable twins are bound to share the disorder or not.

There have just been a couple of twin investigations on BPD, and the discoveries are mixed. The most extensive research done in Norway found that if you have BPD, the odds that your indistinguishable twin has BPD are 35 percent. However, the odds that your twin has BPD are around 7 percent. These discoveries recommend that BPD can be acquired (at any rate somewhat). Some research has shown that BPD might be approximately 50 percent heritable.

Another approach to inspecting whether you can get BPD is to take a gander at BPD rate among first-degree family members of individuals with BPD. The thought here is that if BPD is heritable, and you have BPD, at that point, your parents and relatives have BPD themselves. Discoveries from a couple of studies have demonstrated that somewhere in the range of 10 and 20 percent of first-degree family members of individuals with BPD have BPD as well.

This sounds very low. If the disorder was truly heritable, you may anticipate that most first-degree family members should have it. Consider the general pervasiveness pace of BPD—it's around 1.6 percent. This implies that first-degree family members of individuals with BPD are more than multiple times bound to have BPD than individuals with no connections with people affected by BPD.

BPD and the brain
On the slight off chance that you have BPD, you may have pondered whether your mind in some way or another is unique to the brain of individuals who don't have BPD. You may have seen that you respond distinctively to things than others around you do. You may think strange thoughts, feel stronger feelings, or experience more difficulty preventing yourself from participating in incautious activities. Provided that this is true, you may have pondered whether you essentially have an alternate sort of brain than others do. Notably, it isn't as basic as that. The brain is mind-boggling, with a wide range of

structures and frameworks that collaborate in manners that researchers are simply starting to comprehend. Contrasts in your mind could have been there from birth or even before birth, or they could have been created after some time. Numerous things can impact how the mind works and even how huge certain brain territories are. Brain differences between individuals who have BPD and the individuals who don't have BPD could be of different types. This is not the place to deepen this subject, but your doctor will undoubtedly be able to answer you.

BPD and the environment

As we have talked about, BPD is an unpredictable disorder, and the reasons for BPD are similarly as intricate. A wide range of things needs to be present for somebody to have BPD. Notwithstanding qualities, the mind, and personality, specific beneficial encounters may cause BPD. BPD isn't just about how you were conceived but takes into consideration your background as well.

Nature and nurture

You have likely known about the "nature versus nurture" dispute, which has to do with whether mental disorder is identified with genetic design elements that are available when we are conceived ("nature") or whether they are identified with the environment ("nurture"). In all honesty, this discussion is obsolete. The exploration says that both nature and nurture play a role in every mental disorder. Also, we currently realize that it's not conceivable to isolate character from education— the most recent research shows that the environment can change an individual's qualities.

Nature can likewise impact the action of your mind, the size of specific regions of your brain, and the organic frameworks of your body. Remember this concept as you read on about the natural causes that collaborate with your qualities, mind, and body to cause BPD.

Childhood traumas

The natural factor in BPD that is talked about regularly is youth abuse. Youth abuse is actually what it seems like. Specifically, numerous examinations have shown a connection between BPD and youth sexual maltreatment. Even though the discoveries fluctuate starting with one assessment then onto the next, the best estimate is that about a portion of individuals with BPD have had youth sexual maltreatment.

Could youth sexual maltreatment be one potential reason for BPD? Almost certainly, youth sexual maltreatment, particularly by somebody who should be thinking about the kid (for example, a parent, childcare supplier, or relative), could put somebody in danger for a portion of the disorders that accompany BPD. In addition, a few pieces of research have demonstrated that progressively extreme maltreatment is identified with increasingly serious subjective and relational indications of BPD.

Being too suspicious is another subjective side effect of BPD. On the slight chance that you were explicitly mishandled as a youngster, it wouldn't be astonishing if you experienced disorders to have suspicious thoughts every once in a while. Being somewhat cautious about whom you trust may even help you stay safe on some occasions. The relational side effects that appear to be identified with misuse include, generally, fears of surrender; endeavors to maintain a strategic distance from others; and rough, clamorous connections.

Being mishandled as a youngster can cause you to feel insecure in your associations with others, mainly if the individual who maltreated you was your mom, father, or parental figure. Self-destructive and self-hurt practices likewise appear to be identified with sexual maltreatment. Maybe as anyone might expect, some exploration has discovered that increasingly extreme sexual abuse is identified with progressively serious self-destructive and self-hurt conduct among individuals with BPD.

Is BPD a form of PTSD?
Because of this connection between misuse and BPD, a few people imagine that BPD is an entangled type of post-traumatic stress disorder (PTSD). As we notice in the following pages, PTSD is a turmoil that can be created after somebody encounters an appalling, startling, or incredibly horrendous situation. On the slight off chance that you have PTSD, you may over and over experience memories, recollections, pictures, or dreams of the horrible situation. You may even have flashbacks—clear images of the injury that strike a chord out of the blue and cause you to feel like the occasion is occurring once more. Sexual maltreatment is one sort of horrendous experience that may prompt PTSD.

We don't think that BPD is a type of PTSD, in any case, for several reasons. To start with, around 50 percent of individuals with BPD don't report youth sexual maltreatment, and up to 54 percent of them don't meet the criteria for PTSD. Secondly, a few people with BPD don't report having encountered any awful situation. Tobe diagnosed with PTSD, you have to have faced a seriously distressing encounter. If you haven't had a horrible encounter, you can't have PTSD.

BPD and PTSD in some cases do go connected and can be brought about by similar encounters. However, even if that may be the case, not every person with BPD has PTSD. Hence, we don't feel that BPD is a type of confounded PTSD. PTSD is, by all accounts, a different disorder, even though injury assumes a job in BPD for specific individuals.

Notwithstanding finding out about elements that may have caused BPD in any case, it is significant for you to comprehend what kinds of factors may assist with keeping up BPD after some time. It isn't altogether clear how or why BPD stays for the individuals who have it. However, we accept that a few elements may be engaged with keeping up the disorders identified with BPD.

One such factor might be turbulent or unfriendly life occasions. Individuals with BPD experience an overwhelmingly huge number of unsavory, upsetting circumstances and problems. We have seen individuals who have stopped their occupations more than once a week, had a passing in the family, had a severe auto crash, been deserted by a personal accomplice, tumbled down the stairs, and experienced open mortification. Scientists use the term "persistent emergency" to portray this inclination of individuals with BPD to encounter a colossal number of very distressing occasions. You may have seen this for yourself. You may feel like the emergencies throughout your life never let up. They continue coming, in a steady progression, with no break for you to recover or set yourself up to manage the next catastrophe.

Struggle with others is presumably the most widely recognized factor, and it is a typical trigger of self-hurt and self-destructive conduct among individuals with BPD. Also, some exploration has discovered that being dismissed, fizzling at something, and being separated from everyone else are typical triggers for passionate misery among individuals with BPD. Being continually presented to disordered or unpleasant life occasions may prop your disorders up.

If you are continually under pressure, you may find that you are effectively bothered, genuinely powerless, and experience difficulties adapting to life. Accordingly, you may depend on practices such as self-damage, tranquilize use, or suicide endeavors to cope with reality. In reality, when individuals are upset, they are bound to follow up without much forethought and do things that might be unsafe.

When you are vexed, you are probably going to utilize your assets to dispose of your trouble. This, in any case, leaves not very many assets accessible to prevent yourself from doing imprudent things. Consider how you feel when you are lifting loads: individuals lifting overwhelming loads are bound to drop them when somebody adds another weight or runs out of energy. So also, if you are continually experiencing upsetting life occasions, you may find that your adapting abilities are drained to such an extent that you go to suicide endeavors, self-damage, or medication use.

As you can envision, these sorts of circumstances can get you into an endless loop. First, you experience an extremely unpleasant occasion, and afterward, you feel genuinely bothered. You feel embarrassed, tragic, and perhaps somewhat angry.

If you have BPD, you presumably make some hard memories making sense of how to affect yourself better.

So you resort to something such as self-damage, medications, or alcohol. You feel better after you drink, use medications, or hurt yourself, yet doing these things doesn't assist with taking care of your concern of being dismissed and prompts more disorders and more worry later on. Also, what are you going to do whenever you are worried? You'll likely take part in the same disorder practices that helped you feel better last time, creating this vicious cycle.

Chapter 5

The Course of Borderline Personality Disorder

When battling a mental disorder, it is essential to realize precisely what's in store as the confusion advances. Being diagnosed with a mental disorder can be very startling. To begin with, as we have examined, the general disposition toward individuals with psychological disorders isn't constantly an illuminated one. There is not a great deal of open data on to what extent BPD keeps going. Also, probably the most frightening thing for individuals is not knowing the course of the illness.

Not realizing to what extent you may have BPD or whether it will pass can be genuinely alarming. But, on the other hand, if you somehow managed to be determined to have malignant growth or coronary illness, you would unquestionably need to realize to what extent you ought to anticipate that your sickness should last, how exceptional it may get, which indications are probably going to appear first, and which manifestations or disorders may stay for more time.

Essentially, having data about what's in store as the mental disorder advances and how that issue is probably going to change after some time can remove a portion of the vulnerability and fear of the disease, making it not so much frightening but rather more reasonable to accept.

Likewise, realizing what's in store can assist you with preparing and set you up to adapt better later on.

For every one of these reasons, it is essential to get as much data as possible about the feasible movement of BPD after some time, including the side effect you can hope to change and those that are presumably going to remain. In the relatively recent past, individuals imagined that BPD kept going forever. That is one reason why BPD is known as a "personality disorder."

The essential thought was that if BPD is a piece of somebody's personality, it very well may be relied upon to proceed all through such an individual's reality. Nowadays, we realize that personality disorder is not steady. It is presumably most secure to accept that scatters like BPD will change (or even leave) after some time. The possibility that individuals may recoup from personality disorder is generally new and conflicts with numerous primary fantasies. This is why it is fundamental for you to peruse this section and get precise data about the timetable of recovery from BPD.

Another significant point to remember is that the manifestations of BPD differ in their soundness after some time. A few side effects appear to stay for quite a while, and others may show signs of improvement or may even leave sooner or later. Subsequently, you can expect a few indications to change moderately rapidly, and others may not change by any stretch of the imagination. Knowing which indications may change and which may not change will enable you to comprehend what's in store in your recouping process.

How long it takes to recover from BPD

Albeit psychological wellness experts once believed that BPD was a deep-rooted disorder with minimal possibility of recouping, this conviction depended entirely on poorly established suppositions and recounted proof and had no premise in analytical research.

Indeed, not long ago, there was no analytical research to disclose to us to what extent BPD keeps going. In the course of the most recent few decades, in any case, specialists have started to concentrate on how this disorder disappears after some time, following numerous individuals with this disorder to perceive how and when they recoup. The aftereffects of two such long-haul pieces of research have furnished us with cause for trust. More or less, this examination tells us that once-held convictions about the security and hopelessness of BPD are off-base. In particular, there is currently a ton of proof that many people hospitalized with BPD will never again meet the criteria for this disorder in just six years.

In addition, practically 50% of the previous patients didn't meet the criteria for BPD four years after they got it, and 69 percent, despite everything, didn't meet the criteria for BPD six years after they got it. Indeed, through the span of the six-year time frame, 74 percent of the patients who had begun with BPD never again met the criteria for BPD sooner or later during the examination. Similarly as significant, a great number of people (94 percent) who had quit meeting criteria for BPD never met criteria for BPD again during the remainder of the investigation. Thus, BPD didn't leave to flare back up once more. Instead, for some individuals, it went away for good.

The other significant point to remember is that this examination was not a treatment study, and it was not planned to look at the advantages of a specific treatment for BPD. In this way, even though most patients kept accepting some mental treatment throughout the examination, the sorts of treatment they got fluctuated. Not every person stayed in treatment all through the whole six years. A few people were not in therapy by any means. This is significant because it reveals to us that even without a specific condition of the art treatment for BPD, numerous individuals with BPD will inevitably show signs of improvement after some time.

Another investigation has likewise taken a gander at the course of events for BPD, in correlation with that for three other personality disorders and significant sorrow. In particular, over a large portion of the patients with BPD in their investigation quit meeting criteria for BPD sooner or later inside the initial two years of the examination. Furthermore, if that doesn't sound confident enough, think about this: more than 25 percent of the patients with BPD revealed no manifestations after just a year, indicating a complete recovery. Likewise, this investigation found that 10 percent of patients with BPD quit meeting the criteria for BPD inside the initial half-year of the examination.

Thus, rather than the possibility that BPD some way or another sticks to you like paste, BPD might be more curable than we at any point thought. BPD may even be a pathology with more hope for recouping than some others. For example, disorders like depression and bipolar disorder return ordinarily during an individual's life. Conversely, recovery from BPD regularly implies that it won't return in the future. Thus, that is the uplifting news.

The six-year recovery rate isn't 100 percent; in this manner, it is imperative to see a portion of the things that make a recovery from BPD slower or interfere with healing from BPD.

Therefore, now we should direct our focus toward the things that interfere with recovery from BPD.

Interfering variables

The more disorders you have, the harder it very well may be to address every one of them. For the most part, individuals find that having another mental illness makes recuperation from BPD increasingly more difficult. What's more, specific clutters make it particularly difficult to recoup from BPD.

In the following few pages, we will outline some variables that can make recouping from BPD more difficult.

Substance abuse

One sort of issue that most interferes with recovery from BPD is substance abuse. There are two sorts of substance use disorders:

substance misuse and substance reliance. Substance misuse includes experiencing conditions throughout your life because of alcohol or medication abuse; and substance reliance includes being so engrossed with alcohol or medication utilize that you use them constantly, put everything on the line to get drugs or alcohol, or have a high resilience for drugs or alcohol.

This reveals to us that a substance use disorder drastically interferes with the recouping of BPD. Even though we don't know precisely why this is the situation, substance abuse disorders commonly aggravate individuals' conditions and have many negative results. In addition, a portion of the adverse consequences of substance misuse is fundamentally the same as a portion of the disorders that individuals with BPD battle with.

For instance, substance misuse can prompt hazardous or wild conduct, make individuals progressively passionate, and start disorders when it comes to relationships. Sounds common? Interestingly, numerous individuals with BPD may utilize substances to escape from a portion of these disorders and get brief help from passionate torment. However, over the long haul, substance misuse is likely going to aggravate these disorders as well.

PTSD
Another issue that regularly follows BPD and appears to interferes with recovery is PTSD. As you may recall from previous chapters, PTSD is one of the issues that can happen following the experience of a horrendous situation.

These two disorders regularly are connected because numerous individuals with BPD have encountered horrible situations in their lives, including youth misuse. Along these lines, similar occasions that may make somebody bound to have BPD likewise make somebody bound to have PTSD. Precisely why having PTSD may make it harder to recuperate from BPD isn't known, yet there are a few potential clarifications.

To start with, if you have both PTSD and BPD, the unfortunate encounters you had growing up might cause both disorders. As we have examined, a wide range of sorts of upsetting encounters can prompt BPD. These encounters run from not feeling like you fit in with your family and not considering you need severe physical and sexual maltreatment. In any case, since you can have PTSD on the slight off chance that you have encountered a horrible accident, the odds are that individuals who have both BPD and PTSD had the most severe distressing encounters growing up.

The way that having the two disorders might indicate that you have endured especially troublesome and horrible encounters may clarify why it is more difficult to recoup from BPD. PTSD may interfere with recovery from BPD because the disorders accompanying PTSD are like the disorders we see in BPD. Having "twofold portions" of similar conditions can make it progressively hard to manage those disorders.

In any case, feeling dysregulation is likewise a piece of PTSD. If you have the two disorders, you may anticipate a twofold portion of feeling dysregulation, making it progressively hard to recoup from either condition. The equivalent could be required to happen with the disorder of evasion. Individuals with PTSD will, in general, stay away from the circumstances and thoughts that help them to remember the injury they have encountered. Also, as we have examined, individuals with BPD will, in general, adapt to their feelings by staying away from them. Since evasion may shield you from confronting your disorders head-on, this twofold portion of shirking may make it much harder for you to recoup from BPD.

As discussed in more considerable detail beneath, recuperating from BPD appears to require dynamic critical thinking, and escapism of any kind seems to interfere with progress. Cognitive Behavioral Therapy comes handy in this circumstance as you may imagine by now.

Temperament and BPD

The nearness of temperament and uneasiness disorder, significant discouragement, and frenzy disorder specifically likewise interfere with recovery from BPD. On the slight chance that you have both of these personality disorders, it could imply that you are more genuinely powerless or have considerably more trouble dealing with your feelings than if you had BPD alone.

This could clarify why it would take somewhat longer for you to recoup from BPD. Additionally, much like with PTSD, individuals with other disorders do numerous things to maintain a strategic distance from their feelings. For instance, individuals with an anxiety disorder will, in general, abstain from going places where they know they may have a panic attack. Albeit we all maintain a strategic distance from tension or different feelings on occasion, keeping away from or doing whatever it takes not to feel these feelings can aggravate them.

If you have this disorder, you may have seen that the more you attempt to avoid tension or uneasiness in inciting occasions, the more frightening life becomes. In another case of how mindset and tension disorder may prompt evasion, discouraged individuals will generally pull back and disconnect themselves from others, essentially keeping away from exercises. Thus, discouragement and nervousness disorder may make it harder to recoup from BPD because the evasion that accompanies these clutters fuels the flames of emotional torment and keeps you from doing the very things that would enable you to recover.

Other personalities disorders

The presence of another arrangement of personality disorders likewise appears to interfere with recouping from BPD. In particular, when individuals with BPD additionally meet the criteria for a nervous frightful personality disorder, they are bound to keep on meeting the criteria for BPD following six years.

Individuals with hindered personalities will, in general, be mindful and restless in new circumstances, and they are frequently bashful and not particularly cordial. Things being what they are, how might having an increasingly restrained personality meddle with recovery from BPD? Indeed, recovery from BPD takes a great deal of challenging work. It requires a great deal of vitality and includes a ton of individual hazards. It is simpler to recoup from BPD if you are eager to put yourself in the conditions to succeed.

For individuals brought into the world progressively timid and on edge, it tends to be hard to stir up the nerve and vitality to devote themselves entirely to the healing process. Thus, individuals brought into the world more dynamic and friendly may have an advantage in recouping from BPD. Of course, it doesn't imply that you won't have the option to recuperate from BPD. However, it means that recovery might be increasingly complex for you, and you may need to propel yourself more than others need to. Actually, on the slight chance that you realize that you are timid, use what you have discovered here as your inspiration to be increasingly dynamic and look for the help you need.

Changes across different types of BPD symptoms
The manifestations of BPD fall into five principal classes: passionate, relational, subjective, personality/self, and social. Many people with BPD battle with these zones, having disorders with their feelings, considerations, and connections, and frequently captivating in dangerous practices. A portion of these side effects might be viewed as a component of your personality. For example, you may have been a passionate individual, and you may be an enthusiastic individual. There's nothing wrong with that. The disorder appears to emerge when you do certain things to manage your feelings, for example, utilizing drugs or hurting yourself.

You could consider your emotions a personality quality—a key ingredient in the blend that makes you your identity. If you have an enthusiastic personality, we probably won't say that that should change without question. On the contrary, what you do when annoyed or in an emergency—endeavoring suicide, utilizing medications, or harming yourself—should be bound to change.

These practices are not what your identity is; they are things you may do at the time to adapt to disorders you have.

What does this have to do with BPD? For reasons unknown, specific side effects of BPD change more rapidly than others, and this may have to do with whether the side effects are a piece of your personality or just how you approach your pain. What side effects would you be able to hope to improve the most? As we referenced above, the examination shows that the social side effects of BPD change more than others. For instance, we examined before, just one-fourth of the patients with BPD revealed self-hurt or self-destructive conduct following six years, even though 80 percent had these practices toward the beginning of the examination.

This is an astonishing diminishing number and an excellent sign, given how unsafe these practices are. So also, by the multi-year point, the level of patients manhandling substances was just 25 percent, down from 50 percent. This lets us know that if you have BPD, you can anticipate that your conduct indications should change most rapidly and be decreased through treatment (contrasted with different manifestations of BPD). Then again, if you are determined to have BPD, you most likely ought not to anticipate that your passionate indications should change excessively. As we clarified beforehand, these enthusiastic indications incorporate great sentiments of gloom, sadness, blame, outrage, tension, melancholy, and void. The way that the patients kept on having these feelings may mirror how individuals with BPD are essentially designed to be sincerely extraordinary and to encounter their feelings all the more firmly. Even though these feelings can be excruciating, they don't need to interfere with your life, and, without different troubles, they are not indications of mental disorders.

This discloses that you ought to most likely not anticipate that a portion of your emotional side effects should change to such an extent and ought not to view yourself or your treatment as a disappointment if they don't work as you expect.

These feelings may stay with you for an extended period, and they don't need to shield you from having the quality of life you desire. This doesn't imply that you will continually feel as awful as you do now or that you will consistently be in as much enthusiastic pain. Instead, we think that the more you figure out how to control your coping practices, deal with your relationships, and build up the existence you need, the better you will feel over time.

The point we are attempting to make here is twofold. In the first place, everybody encounters negative feelings. It is beyond the realm of imagination to expect to be human and alive and never feel tragic, restless, furious, lonely, etc. To be human means to feel feelings, and a considerable lot of these feelings are negative. We just genuinely need to accept that individuals will consistently have negative emotions even with the best and most sophisticated treatment since this is a piece of being alive.

We need to make the other point that a few people are brought into the world in more extreme circumstances than others. Therefore, they feel things more emphatically and experience their feelings more seriously.

This is only how they are, a piece of their personality. Furthermore, since it is a piece of their character, this is most likely not change. In this way, if you are more genuinely extraordinary than others are, you are most likely to continue going to feel things more strongly than others. Also, that is not a terrible thing and doesn't need to hurt your quality of life in any capacity. It's simply unrealistic to dispose of your feelings, and attempting to do that is a useless fight.

Plus, we believe that getting your practices leveled out and learning better approaches for adapting to your disorders will cause you to feel better and assist you with having the existence you need. Along these lines, by concentrating your vitality on changing how you adapt to your feelings and the disorders throughout your life, you will presumably see preferable outcomes over you would on the slight off chance that you attempted to change a piece of your personality or disposition. The pace of progress for disorders with considerations and connections falls somewhere close to that for social and passionate side effects. A portion of these manifestations appears to change before long, and others seem to be increasingly similar to the enthusiastic side effects of BPD.

Among the subjective indications, severe types of neurotic reasoning changed the most over six years. Yet, different kinds of considerations and dissociative manifestations remained genuinely average. Concerning relational side effects, the ones that changed the most rapidly were the conduct side effects we discussed previously, appearing as rash practices inside relationships.

These side effects included severe challenges with advisors, insecure and stormy relationships, and the propensity to put outrageous requests on others. These indications presumably cause many disorders in individuals' lives. Thus it is excellent news that they appear to improve in a short period. Then again, other relational side effects have a passionate segment, similar to fears of relinquishment and challenges enduring being separated from everyone else. Thus they will, in general, stick around for more extended periods.

The following is a preview of the side effects that are well on the way to improve after some time.

- severe suspicious reasoning;
- unstable, stormy connections;
- the propensity to put extraordinary requests on others.

Here is a list of the manifestations that improve over more extended periods.

- Wretchedness;
- nervousness;
- outrage;
- bitterness;
- blame;
- dissociative episodes;
- negative convictions about oneself or the world;
- fears of being separated from everyone else.

Chapter 6

Problems Connected to Borderline Personality Disorder

As we have examined all through this book, the side effects of BPD are troubling. Individuals who experience the ill effects of this disorder regularly feel like they are crazy.

They may feel as though their feelings are their enemies, filling no other need than to make their lives hopeless. Having such overpowering feelings, considerations, practices, and relational connections are sufficient to make life a battle. Tragically, numerous individuals with BPD have to battle other mental illnesses and issues. In the following pages, we will give you an overview of the mental disorders that can follow BPD.

Mental disorders that can follow BPD

BPD is followed by different disorders. Many people with BPD have one other mental disorder, and some of them have a few different conditions. On the slight off chance that you have BPD, you may have seen that, notwithstanding this disorder, you likewise have disorders like sadness or uneasiness or battle with alcohol or medication abuse. As we referenced previously, adapting to the indications of various mental diseases can be a significant test, and it can make recuperating from BPD increasingly troublesome. Subsequently, it is critical to comprehend the disorders that frequently follow BPD.

Substance abuse

Substance misuse and reliance are fundamental among individuals with BPD. Studies have discovered that upwards of 66% of individuals with BPD additionally have substance use disorders, and roughly one-fifth of individuals who misuse substances meet the criteria for BPD.

Emotional pain

The intuitive response to this inquiry may lie in the entirely justifiable want to stay away from passionate torment. Simply put, substances give a break from emotional suffering. As we examined previously, needing to evade or avoid upsetting feelings is typical for those who suffer from BPD. The more significant part of us don't begin the day saying, "I know this day is loaded with nervousness!" or "I can hardly wait for seven days brimming with grief!" Yet, when we are vexed, we frequently need to escape from those emotions as fast as we can.

One approach to escaping from these emotions is to dodge whatever it is that is causing us trouble. For instance, when individuals are miserable, they may call a companion to take their psyche off their bitterness. When individuals are on edge, they may count to ten or take full breaths to get away from their tension. At the point when individuals are angry, they may leave the circumstance that is driving them mad. These models paint a clear picture: when we experience upsetting or awkward feelings, we frequently need to escape from these emotions and the circumstances that bring them up.

Escaping emotional pain

Even though the longing to evade enthusiastic trouble is ordinary, a few disorders accompany maintaining a strategic distance from or getting away from awkward feelings. One of these is that keeping away from your sentiments doesn't assist you with managing the disorders that prompted these emotions in any case. For example, have you at any point wound up feeling truly disturbed about something and afterward doing your best to abstain from feeling this way? For example, suppose that you got a busy working schedule and your supervisor said that you need to begin showing up at work prior and accomplishing your work more productively.

At the point when you heard this, you felt upset—possibly miserable, on edge, or even somewhat embarrassed about your performance. If you, at that point, totally stayed away from these sentiments by utilizing medications or drinking each morning before work, you may feel somewhat better at the time. However, you would not stand a chance in keeping your job. Nonetheless, you focused on how you were feeling and thought about how to accomplish better results. As a result, you may show signs of improvement over a relatively short period. As should be obvious, one issue with evading feelings (mainly through medications) is that it prevents you from confronting and taking care of your disorders.

Your disorders stay, making you progressively agitated, and you get trapped in an endless loop of maintaining a strategic distance from problems while your conditions keep on accumulating. Another issue with keeping away from feelings is identified with the way that individuals with BPD will, in general, be more enthusiastic than others are. As we've said before, there's nothing wrong with being a passionate individual. Indeed, if you are enthusiastic, you may carry on a more extravagant and fuller life than individuals who aren't as passionate.

Accordingly, you may once in a while end up in trouble for how you manage your emotions. We imagine that is the reason a few people with BPD resort to substance misuse. Consider it: substances (for example, alcohol, weed, recommended medications, or heroin) cause individuals to enter a modified state of consciousness—a psychological state wherein you don't feel like yourself. You may feel increasingly secure, upbeat, quiet, or numb. As a general rule, individuals with BPD use substances to seek temporary help from extreme emotions and thoughts that are hard to endure. However, the keyword here is temporary. What happens next is not a secret at all.

Alcohol, drugs and BPD

A significant disorder with utilizing substances to escape is that this departure is exceptionally fleeting, and a short time later, you may feel far more terrible than you did before taking the substance. Essentially, the very thing you used to cause yourself to feel better winds up making you feel considerably worse later on. What do you believe you're going to need to do when you feel more terrible? Utilize more medications or alcohol! That is the issue.

Another issue is that the more you use medications and alcohol, the more you develop resistance to these substances. Therefore, you need a more significant dose of your picked substance to get a similar impact in the long run. For example, when you were eighteen and exploring different avenues regarding alcohol, two beers may have been sufficient to get you drunk. Nowadays, you may require a six-pack to get a similar impact.

Also, you may encounter withdrawal symptoms on the slight off chance that you utilize a substance sufficiently long. These are the body's response to not having the substance, regularly followed by a craving for the substance and awkward physical feelings (fomentation, nervousness, sweating, and sickness, among others). When this begins occurring, individuals may start to utilize medications and alcohol basically to dispose of the withdrawal side effects themselves.

Now, the substance starts to control the individual's life. Relationships may be compromised, deadlines at work may not be met, and medical issues may arise. With these negative results, for what reason would anybody keep on utilizing these substances? The transitory help that substances give can be extraordinary so that individuals in outrageous enthusiastic torment might be happy to give up the long-term adverse outcomes.

Eating disorders

Dietary problems are likewise very typical among people with BPD. Studies have discovered that upwards of 50 percent of individuals with BPD have a dietary issue. For the most part, nutritional disorders appear as either anorexia (limiting nourishment admission to such an extent that the individual is seriously underweight) or bulimia. Similar to the case with substance use disorders, there are some valid reasons why many individuals with BPD battle with a dietary illness.

The primary explanation is like the one we talked about above regarding substance use disorders, and it is generally appropriate for bulimia. Like substance use, both eating and vomiting can adapt to enthusiastic pain and alleviate negative feelings. Consider it—eating is one of the most widely recognized ways individuals relieve stress. Indeed, even individuals who don't have a dietary disorder frequently use nourishment to give comfort during times of pressure or pain.

How frequently have you or has somebody you know gone to food for comfort when feeling down, pitiful, lonely, or upset? Without a doubt, clinical specialists have recommended that the inclination for individuals to utilize nourishment for solace may help clarify the high paces of weight in the United States. Much like with substances, the longing to use nutrition to help may even have a natural premise. Specific sorts of foods, for example, pieces of bread, cakes, chips, treats, and candies (the very kinds of food sources that individuals tend to binge on), can improve your mood, prompting transitory well-being, comfort, and a general feeling of tranquility.

Eating these sugary or greasy foods takes a shot at the "happy part" of your brain, causing the secretion of dopamine, like the impacts of certain medications. In this way, it isn't astonishing that, in the same way as healthy people, individuals with BPD frequently resort to foods to calm themselves and mitigate their troubles. Unfortunately, however, even in this case, even though gorging can give impermanent alleviation from passionate torment, it can turn into a dependence after some time.

Fundamentally, the more individuals eat to adapt to their feelings, the more they have to eat to get the equivalent enthusiastic help—prompting an ever-increasing number of binge sessions, just as an expanding feeling of being wild. Furthermore, if you have bulimia, the more you eat, the more you will want to cleanse (by spewing, taking diuretics, or practicing unreasonably training sessions). However, cleansing is highly hazardous and can prompt significant medical disorders. Additionally, it doesn't work. Some researches have demonstrated that vomiting after a dinner disposes of just around 33% of the injected calories.

Thus, this eating pattern to manage feelings and cleansing to maintain a strategic distance from weight gain is an awful one that can assume control over your life. Sooner or later, a few people find that they begin to invest practically the entirety of their energy, vomiting what they just ate. Also, to add to the addictive idea of bulimia, cleansing can give transitory alleviation from passionate agony, as individuals once in a while experience an arrival of strain or serenity following a cleansing. Unfortunately, this help can be solid to such an extent that it makes individuals progressively inclined to overeating then vomiting later on, regardless of the probable damages to their relationships, well-being, and lives.

Body shaming

A second explanation that dietary disorders are typical among individuals with BPD may have to do with body shaming. Even though nutritional disorders are not exclusively the consequence of a poor self-perception or desire to be skinny, the vast majority with dietary problems are disappointed with their bodies and aversion to how they look. Since numerous individuals with BPD have had negative encounters, it isn't extraordinary for them to have encountered psychological mistreatment.

What's more interesting, though, is that one type of psychological mistreatment may enforce negative judgments about an individual's looks of themselves. If you experienced childhood in a family where you were encouraged to be fat, you might have grown up loathing everything about yourself. One thing about ourselves that can be particularly simple to hate in our society is our bodies. Surrounding us, we get the message that it is ideal to be skinny. If you grew up loathing yourself and your body, you might be significantly bound to get tied up with the message that a skinny body is a perfect body. The practices accompanying dietary disorders—cleansing and confining nourishment admission—can be an individual's sensational endeavors to change their body shape and weight because of body disappointment.

Need of control

Something that can generally be upsetting for individuals is an absence of control. On the slight chance that you have BPD, you may feel like your life, feelings, connections, and practices are wild. Accordingly, you may feel urgent to discover some method for controlling, at any rate, a little piece of your life. A dietary problem like anorexia might be typical among individuals with BPD because this disorder can give individuals an essential feeling of control.

Even though this feeling of control is a fantasy since dietary problems, for the most part, take on their very own existence and become crazy, intentionally limiting nourishment admission and deciding not to eat can furnish individuals with a transitory feeling of authority over probably some part of their lives. Indeed, it's likely not a coincidence that refuting to eat is something that the vast majority would discover extremely difficult to do. People need nourishment to live, and it is an essential human impulse to eat until feeling full. When individuals don't eat enough, they can feel powerless, and tired, and they can experience issues while working. In this way, it is hard to forgo eating persistently.

This is what makes consuming fewer calories so troublesome. In any case, limiting food intake can cause somebody to feel like they are highly grounded and in charge. This can be a severe consoling encounter when your life feels wild. Once more, the disorder is that this control isn't genuine and that severe nourishment limitation can become dangerous. In any case, the longing to have power and apply this over one's life is reasonable and an essential human need. Just find something positive to exercise your control. Otherwise, you will do more harm than good.

Melancholy

Numerous individuals with BPD likewise experience sorrow. Discouragement is something beyond misery. Depression is presumably one of the most widely recognized scatters found among individuals with BPD. Researchers have discovered that 41 to 87 percent of individuals with BPD additionally battle with sadness.

To comprehend why discouragement is so common among individuals with BPD, we should audit the side effects of BPD. Individuals with BPD frequently have troublesome relationships, described by arguments, breakups, and even maltreatment. What's more important, though, is that numerous individuals with BPD have extreme feelings of trepidation that they will be left alone. Individuals with BPD experience negative feelings much of the time and may feel there is nothing they can do to adapt to these feelings. They might not have quite a sense of their identity, and they may stress that others are talking over them behind their backs or are not there for them. This is also a reason why treatments for BPD might be troublesome and agonizing procedures.

At the point when you take a gander at all of these indications together, you can likely observe why somebody with BPD could begin to feel discouraged. The manifestations you experience might be so extreme and long-standing that you may feel that there is nothing that can support you. You may likewise start to accept that there is no reason to keep going. Furthermore, you may begin to feel truly alone because of stormy relationships and consistent battling with the individuals around you. Essentially, the disorders that accompany BPD are regularly the specific fixings that can prompt wretchedness. If a downturn is for sure a reaction to having BPD, you may anticipate that your downturn should diminish once you recoup from BPD, and you would be correct.

Uneasiness disorders

Notwithstanding temperament disorders like misery, BPD is frequently joined by tension disorder. There are many tension disorders. The most widely recognized uneasiness disorder found among individuals with BPD is social tension disorder, alarm disorder, and PTSD.

For instance, researchers have discovered that one-quarter of individuals with BPD likewise experience social tension disorder, 33% to one-half additionally experience an anxiety disorder, and roughly one-half likewise experience PTSD. In the following pages, we will discuss potential reasons why every one of these three uneasiness disorders may be so common among individuals with BPD.

Social anxiety disorder

To begin with, how about we investigate social uneasiness disorder, which includes exceptional apprehensions of being contrarily assessed in social circumstances. For instance, individuals with this disorder may fear to give a speech in front of individuals inspired by a paranoid fear of mortifying themselves. They may likewise fear other social circumstances as well. For example, they meet new individuals, eat in front of other individuals, or go to parties. Because of these feelings, individuals with social anxiety disorder regularly maintain a strategic distance from these circumstances.

Essentially, because of upsetting, troublesome, even harsh encounters, individuals with BPD may get on edge around others and be reluctant to convey their considerations and emotions. Accordingly, they might not have a great deal of trust in relational circumstances. Furthermore, a few hypotheses of the reasons for BPD stress concern possible youth-related traumas. On the slight off chance that you had discrediting encounters over and over, you may get terrified of communicating around others. You may even turn out to be less trusting of others, and you could feel tension when being in social circumstances, particularly circumstances where others may examine you.

Before we dive deeper into how BPD might be related to anxiety disorder, it is significant that we initially give somewhat more insight concerning how this disorder is created. Our bodies are designed to react rapidly to stressful circumstances. Called the "fight-or-flight" reaction, this is essentially a survival tool of our mind.

At the point when we are confronted with danger (real or imaginary), our body sets us up to either battle or escape the circumstance. You will realize this reaction is turned on when you start to notice a fast heartbeat, heavy breath, "limited focus" (where your consideration gets concentrated on just a single thing— like escaping a frightening circumstance), muscle strain, and quick flow of thoughts. Your body is getting ready for a move.

Once more, this is a typical reaction. Some of the time, this reaction can be scary. At the point when we are apprehensive or haven't been dealing with ourselves, our fight-or-flight framework may fire without reason. This would be known as an attack of anxiety. Since there is no danger present, the attack of anxiety appears as though it comes "out of nowhere," and, in this manner, it tends to be alarming.

Individuals who have panic attacks may feel that they are having a coronary failure, going insane, or falling. In any case, an attack of anxiety doesn't mean any of these things. Instead, it presumably implies that you are worried, have not been dealing with yourself so well, and are frightened of being restless. At the point when these things consolidate, the scarcest twinge of anything, in any event, can set off a chain response of increasingly more dread and excitement until, in the long run, you have an attack of anxiety. Episodes of anxiety that happen with no notice are alarming because they are unusual. Individuals essentially don't react well to things that are unusual and unexpected.

Also, this incorporates feelings like frenzy and dread. We can realize when to expect certain emotions and the sorts of things that may make us feel in a certain way, and we are afraid when feelings hit us without reason. Numerous individuals abstain from going places that they think may be hard to escape from on the slight off chance that they begin to have an anxiety attack (for example, a shopping center a long way from home). Others refuse to leave their homes because of fears about having an episode of anxiety in a new place.

This sort of behavior can get so outrageous that individuals may decline to go out by any means. This is called agoraphobia. So how does this all apply to BPD? Just as a result of the idea of BPD and its side effects, individuals who have this disorder may encounter uplifted degrees of stress. If you have BPD, you are most likely more upsetting than others' relationships.

Truth be told, as we referenced in chapter 3, your life, all in all, might be increasingly distressing. Additionally, because individuals with BPD frequently experience disorders dealing with their feelings, your feelings may feel crazy, excessively serious, and unusual.

This will likely build your feelings of anxiety and interfere with your capacity to adapt to everyday life. In this way, your body's fight-or-flight reaction may cause failure to fire, and you may have an attack of anxiety. Researchers recommend that enthusiastic challenges and the pressure related to having these troubles improve the probability that somebody will have an episode of anxiety.

If an anxiety attack happens once, this will prompt stresses and fears over future episodes of anxiety, just as evasion of any circumstance or experience could prompt another attack. Since individuals with BPD as of now tend to keep away from trouble instead of adapting to them, an individual with BPD might be significantly bound to utilize evasion practices because of fits of anxiety. Be that as it may, as we have discussed previously, even though evasion might be compelling at first, it is unquestionably connected with longer-term adverse outcomes.

Chapter 7

Suicidal Behavior and Self-Harm

Suicide and self-hurt are huge issues for individuals with BPD. That is the reason we chose to dedicated a specific chapter just to these subjects. These practices are not exclusively popular among individuals with BPD, but they are probably the most significant disorders that individuals with BPD battle with. Dissimilar to many different diseases that accompany BPD, self-hurt and self-destructive practices are dangerous and extreme consequences.

For this reason, it is fundamental for you to know as much as possible about these practices. Later on, in chapters 11 and 12, we depict a few aptitudes that may assist you with managing considerations about suicide and control your feelings. Here, we give you some data on self-hurt and self-destructive practices, including why individuals once in a while take part in these practices.

The meaning behind bad thoughts

This is a substantially complicated subject. Indeed, even individuals who study and commit self-destructive and self-hurt practices don't generally know how they reach that point when they begin to consider these practices.

Suicide attempts

For an episode to be known as a suicide endeavor, it must be finished with the reasonable expectation to cause death, even though this distinction may appear straightforward.

For example, individuals at times appear at the crisis room after having cut themselves to feel much better and are marked as dangerous for themselves. This misconception may lead an ER specialist to attempt to hospitalize them or put them on a twenty-four-hour mental hold out of fear that they could kill themselves. Even though this may be a smart thought if an individual was really in danger of cutting themselves, it's not helpful if the individual was attempting to get some help and honestly wouldn't like to take their life.

On the other side, here and there, individuals hurt themselves and honestly would like to commit suicide yet are classified as "self-harmers" and are ignored. Right now, those who are in urgent need of help at times don't get the help they need—which can result in fatal consequences. As far as we can tell, there is a significant contrast between harming yourself to murder yourself and harming yourself to feel better. In this manner, you need to know if you are developing this sort of thought or not.

A couple of words and expressions are used to portray self-hurt and self-destructive practices that we find worth mentioning.

- Suicide signal;
- Cry for help;
- Manipulative behavior.

As you read this chapter, you may be asking why individuals with BPD are at such a high risk of hurting themselves. Given what we just said, we have a couple of thoughts regarding why individuals hurt themselves.

Many studies have asked individuals for what reason they hurt themselves, and the most widely recognized explanation that individuals give is that they were attempting to get away or keep away from bad feelings. This is true particularly for individuals with BPD.

For example, in one research, ladies with BPD were asked why they hurt themselves or endeavored suicide. Of these ladies, 96 percent said they occupied with purposeful self-hurt to get away from their feelings; 86 percent said they had made a suicide endeavor to alleviate their feelings. As we have talked about, individuals with BPD are looking for a way to get away from their feelings, and self-harm seems like a viable option.

They have extraordinary feelings that may now and again feel overpowering or unbearable. Simultaneously, they have gigantic trouble dealing with their feelings, and frequently they haven't figured out how to affect themselves better when they are vexed. If you have BPD, you may have seen that you have practically no clue how to make yourself feel better when you are genuinely disturbed. During these occasions, you may be so overpowered by your unique feelings that you begin thinking about some way—any way—that could give you some alleviation.

For specific individuals, one of these ways might be intentional self-hurt. Some exploration has demonstrated that individuals with BPD are more likely than individuals without BPD to report to feel genuinely better after they hurt themselves. Different examinations have seen what happens physiologically (or in the body) when individuals envision harming themselves. For reasons that are still unknown, individuals who have routinely harmed themselves in the past show lower enthusiastic excitement when they envision hurting themselves. Essentially, even though self-hurt has a lot of drawbacks and some actual adverse results, the truth of the matter is that it can cause individuals to feel vastly better at the time.

Even though we accept that the entirety of self-hurt's drawbacks certainly exceeds its transient advantages, the alleviation produced by this conduct strengthens it. It makes individuals depend on it to adapt to passionate torment. Anyway, shouldn't something be said about suicide endeavors? For what reason would suicide help you with getting away from enthusiastic suffering? Indeed, as per one hypothesis, when individuals experience an upsetting occasion, they become concentrated on approaches to feel much better. They can turn out to be so centered on how they may approach feeling better that they can't do much else.

They may begin to experience difficulty focusing and thinking, and, at last, they can get confused in their journey to figure out how to feel much better. If they believe that nothing will ever improve in the future, they may begin imagining that the only way to feel better is to end it all. Again, on the slight off chance that you have BPD and have battled with self-destructive ideas, this may sound commonplace to you.

What you can do about this
Halting self-hurt is most likely as hard for specific individuals to stop smoking for smokers.

Here's one step that you can take right now. Whenever you need to hurt yourself or endeavor suicide, stop and think for a minute. What might you get from it? Consider your purposes behind harming yourself or endeavoring suicide. Frequently, clearing your thoughts is a great way to feel better.

In any case, we advise you to talk to your doctor if these thoughts do not stop. Once again, your doctor is the only one to help you out truly, and this book serves no medical purpose.

Chapter 8

Finding Help for Borderline Personality Disorder

Imagining that you (or somebody you love) may have BPD can welcome many feelings, from fear to anger to sadness. Even though there is help for BPD, discovering this assistance can be an overwhelming encounter. It isn't in every case clear where to turn or what choices to listen to. In this chapter, we will give you some tips to find help as fast as possible.

Internet resources for BPD

The Internet is undoubtedly a resource with regards to information on BPD. Albeit a few sites are beneficial, giving data on accessible medications, different places are full of falsehood, legends, and awful guidance. Clearing your path through the field of alternatives can be highly overwhelming, and it tends to be difficult to tell whom to trust or where to turn to.

The Internet can probably be the best wellspring of data on BPD—as long as you most likely are aware of where to look and visit legitimate and dependable sites. Notwithstanding, there are numerous different methods for discovering data on BPD and countless other assets you can use as you continue looking for help. For instance, a few people find that it is helpful to read books on BPD.

Your neighborhood book shop or library presumably has a variety of books on BPD, including self-improvement guides, collections of memoirs of individuals who have battled with BPD, and reference books composed for specialists or advisors. Depending on what sort of data you are keen on, any of these kinds of books may be helpful to you. Another viable method to acquire data is to converse with a nearby brain science teacher. If you are an understudy, educators in the brain research division at your nearby college may have the option to give you data on BPD or suggest advisors in the region who treat patients with BPD.

You may likewise need to go to a network or college psychological well-being group. Places like these regularly have pamphlets, freebies, or other instructive materials accessible on a broad scope of mental disorders. Furthermore, regardless of whether they don't, somebody who works there may have the option to advise you somewhere else in your local area where you could discover the data you're looking for. Finally, a different method to find information on BPD or get referrals to clinicians or treatment programs is to ask a specialist in BPD. Specialists in similar fields regularly know each other. In this manner, if you discover the name of somebody in your area who treats BPD, you could contact that individual and request that they give you the contact of an expert or a treatment program.

Different types of treatments

Two primary sorts of medicines are accessible for individuals with BPD: mental medications and drugs Cognitive treatments typically include meeting with an emotional wellness expert (for example, once every week) and discussing the sorts of issues you battle with, making sense of where your problems originate from and chipping away at making the sorts of life changes you need to make.

In coming chapters, we will disclose to you significantly increasingly around two specific mental medications that have been seen as extremely accommodating for individuals with BPD. Remember that there are numerous types of cognitive medicines accessible that appear to help.

Treatments ordinarily include:
- Meeting with a specialist.
- Getting an assessment to figure out what kind of drug may work for you.
- Accepting a solution.

You would then meet with the therapist regularly to screen how you are getting along on the drug and any reaction you might be encountering (It would be ideal if you see chapter 10 for more subtleties of taking drugs medicines). In the following few pages, we talk about the sorts of mental and prescription medications that you may use in your endeavors to find help.

Mental treatments

Contingent upon where you live, there might be an assortment of treatment choices accessible for BPD. Frequently, these medications will vary as far as how exceptional they are and to what extent they last. Ordinarily, more-escalated drugs have a shorter span than less concentrated medicines. There are also hospitalization programs.

These projects include short stays (in some cases as fast as one day, and typically just a couple of days). Hospitalization treatment programs are commonly utilized when individuals are in an emergency or at genuine risk of murdering themselves. Regularly, the goal of this sort of treatment is to assist individuals enduring an immediate crisis. The drawback of hospitalization treatments is that it removes individuals from their ordinary lives for some time.

Furthermore, even though escaping from your life may seem like quite a beneficial thing to you, it tends to be an issue since it keeps individuals from truly managing their challenges. Since this kind of treatment is so concentrated, it is typically not prescribed for expanded time frames. Usually, specialists suggest what is known as a partial hospitalization program.

These programs usually include a few hours of treatment each day, for a few days every week. Since individuals return home around evening time and are not under direct supervision twenty-four hours a day, these projects are regularly used to assist individuals in transitioning from a hospitalization program to a more independent form of treatment. Incomplete emergency clinic programs are getting increasingly well-known and are accessible in numerous hospitals. In addition, there are many halfway emergency clinic programs that give particular medicines to individuals with BPD. The least escalated and most popular sort of treatment is outpatient care. For many people, at-home treatment includes somewhere in the range of one to five hours of therapy for each week.

Regularly, this sort of treatment comprises individual treatment for a couple of meetings for each week, which might be joined with some gathering treatment or cooperation in a care group. A wide range of sorts of individual therapy might be accessible where you are. The following are the most famous particular treatment out there.

- Cognitive-behavioral treatment. This sort of treatment assists individuals with learning new abilities for dealing with their feelings, musings, or practices. CBT is regularly a genuinely organized type of treatment, with meetings concentrating on making sense of examples that aren't working well overall, learning new aptitudes, and changing practices that are not valuable. Likewise, CBT includes homework assignments, where customers practice new abilities and change practices outside of treatment meetings.

- Dialectical behavioral treatment (DBT). DBT is a unique kind of CBT that consolidates the components of CBT that we discussed before. We will cover DBT much better in the coming chapters.

- Psycho-dynamic treatment. This sort of treatment assists individuals with making sense of why they do the things they do and where these examples originate from. Psycho-dynamic treatments center a great deal around individuals' encounters growing up, helping them perceive how past meetings with parental figures and others impact how they act today. There is a wide range of sorts of psycho-dynamic treatments, going from more to less organized and from more to less expensive. Psycho-dynamic medicines are less organized than CBT and are less inclined to learn new adapting abilities and do homework outside of the meeting.

Albeit every one of these various sorts of medications can be helpful, specialists on the treatment of BPD frequently state that it is ideal for picking the least-concentrated treatment conceivable. Fundamentally, the more your treatment can be coordinated into your reality, the happier you will be.

Medical treatments

Notwithstanding these various kinds of mental treatments, certain medicines may help ease a portion of BPD indications. Specialists in the treatment of BPD, for the most part, agree that it is ideal to utilize drugs in combination with mental medications since prescriptions alone don't appear to work. For the most part, individuals observe a therapist for prescription treatment, albeit some essential consideration doctors will likewise recommend mental medicines.

Various kinds of emotional well-being experts can give mental appraisals and medications to BPD, including clinical analysts (psychological wellness experts in clinical brain research), specialists (clinical specialists with preparation in the treatment of mental issues), and social laborers (psychological wellness experts with an MSW or LICSW).

These kinds of emotional well-being experts are allowed to prescribe mental medicines. Always remember that only specialists can give prescription medications.

Mental assessment

When you get an intensive mental assessment, you can hope to be posed many questions about your state of mind, feelings, musings, and dangerous practices. A ton of the questions will concentrate on the sorts of side effects you are managing now, and some will get information about things you may have endured for a significant amount of time.

A mental assessment may likewise incorporate filling out a few forms or surveys about things like your temperament, personal history, current situations, clinical history, and current drugs.

A few people have a ton of trouble opening up and offering individual data to another person— particularly somebody they have quite recently met. If you are dealing with this issue, you may be terrified that the individual leading your assessment will pass judgment on you, dismiss you, abuse your secrecy by telling others everything about you, or even conclude that you are insane and hospitalize you. We recommend that you express them to the expert you are meeting with if you have any of these worries. Mention to this individual what your stresses and concerns are. At that point, when you have gotten some consolation, be as transparent as conceivable about yourself and your challenges. The primary way you can find support for your issues is if the expert you are meeting with has exact data about your problems.

Singular treatment

Numerous individual specialists will likewise be keen on finding out about your past, including what your initial associations with loved ones resembled, what your close connections (assuming any) have been similar to, and how you did in school. Your specialist may likewise need to find out about your relatives (counting whether they have any psychological well-being issues or judgments and whether they are in treatment). When your specialist has found out about your present issues and some of what you have experienced previously, they will presumably need to build up a treatment contract with you—at the end of the day, an understanding about your goals for treatment and the focal point of your meetings. Most specialists have a conversation with their patients about their treatment goals, what they might want to achieve, or what direction they want to move towards during the treatment.

This conversation is expected to ensure that the specialist and patient concede to the focal point of treatment and comprehend the treatment goals. When this understanding is reached, treatment will continue. However, as we talked about previously, the real focal point of treatment and structure of the meetings will rely upon the kind of treatment.

Group therapy

Since group treatments are so various and have various goals and purposes, this type of therapy will be much different if compared to individual therapy. For instance, it can vary upon the specific sort of group treatment you are taking part into. If you are joining a skill-based group, you will likely be asked to present yourself to the group's participants quickly. Afterward, the group mediator will go ahead with the material for that day. If you are joining a relational or psycho-dynamic group, the presentations might be increasingly formal, and you might be asked to give more data about yourself and for what reason you are joining the therapy group. In this instance, other individuals will likely provide much more information about themselves as well. Or on the other hand, if you are beginning another group treatment, with every new part contributing to the group, the primary meeting may include longer presentations marginally from all the individuals of the group and the group chiefs, and a conversation of the principles and rules for being in the group.

Prescription treatments

Even though this isn't generally the situation, if you are seeing somebody get drugs, you can most likely expect that the meetings will be fewer and shorter. Even though a principal couple of meetings with a specialist might be longer and include getting familiar with your present and past side effects and medications, later meetings might be just fifteen to thirty minutes. These meetings will most likely concentrate principally on your present side effects, any adjustments in side effects you have encountered, and any reactions of the medicines you have taken note of.

All in all, if you are seeing somebody just for drugs, the focal point of the gatherings with this individual will be on issues identified with the medicines, instead of on different topics you might be managing by yourself. That being said, many people who give drug medications have been prepared to provide mental medicines. Along these lines, if you don't have an individual specialist and are seeing somebody for drug treatment only, we would urge you to approach this individual for help when you are battling with your demons, even if you did not get in contact with them for this reason in the first place.

The help of a doctor is always a valuable resource during difficult times, do not be afraid to take advantage of it.

Chapter 9

Dialectal Behavioral Therapy

As we have referenced all through this book, there is hope for those who battle with BPD. There are viable medications for BPD— medicines that assist individuals with figuring out how to lessen crazy conduct, reach their goals, and improve their lives in essential areas. Dialectal Behavior Therapy is one of two or three mental medicines that have been seen as valuable for individuals with BPD.

Persuasive behavioral therapy: building a life worth living

DBT isn't a "quit attempting to execute yourself" treatment; instead, it includes helping individuals create lives that are worth living. These goals (having an actual existence worth living and halting self-destructive conduct) go hand in hand. It is difficult to want to live if your life seems not worth living, and it is difficult to build up an actual existence worth living if you attempt to end it.

There are a few entryways in the room; you can't see them. One of the entryways has a black-out light underneath it. This is the "suicide entryway." The suicide entryway is enticing— it's simpler to see than different entryways, and you happen to know the path to it. Along these lines, you invest your energy stayed outdoors at the suicide entryway, on occasion merely taking a gander at it and feeling support by the possibility that there's an exit plan. The issue is that when you hang out at the suicide entryway, you can't see different entrances that lead out of the dim room and into an actual existence worth living.

Another issue with strolling through the suicide entryway is that you genuinely have no clue what is behind it. Experiencing that entryway resembles bouncing into a pool when you have no clue whether it is brimming with water or completely dry cement. Nobody comprehends what you will discover when you go through that door! We genuinely have no clue what happens to individuals who execute themselves. Nobody has.

A few people feel that suicide offers harmony or a getaway from their issues, yet imagine a scenario where this isn't true. It's a substantial hazard to take. Consider the possibility that you executed yourself because your partner left you just to discover that you were bound to an unfathomable length of time of being rejected by your partner again and again. At that point, you'd be in a challenging situation since you couldn't execute yourself to escape being dead! DBT centers around assisting individuals with BPD locate different entryways out of the dim room and into the light of an actual existence that is satisfying, charming, fulfilling, and — to the exclusion of everything else—worth living.

The beginning of DBT

All things considered, before DBT tagged along, the shame of BPD was far more terrible than it currently is. Individuals had no clue how to treat people with BPD. What's more frustrating is that something generally unpleasant for specialists is not having the option to support their patients effectively.

Individuals discover these intriguing thoughts and recollect them. In developing DBT, we thought of many ideas that appear to be adhering to a significant number of the clinicians, scientists, and customers who have found out about DBT.

Figuring out how to build up an actual existence worth living includes making sense of how to oversee and endure feelings, control practices, focus on the present moment, and explore associations with others. In addition, advisors must be caring and non-judgmental, and they should adjust acknowledgment of the customer by helping the customer roll out significant improvements throughout everyday life. Individuals with BPD are doing as well as expected, but they need to change for the better.

Out of nowhere, advisors assisting individuals with BPD had a lot of thoughts regarding how to help individuals with this issue—ideas that adhered to them like paste and made specialists keen on treating patients with BPD.

Feeling vulnerability includes three aspects.

- emotional softness;
- emotional reactivity;
- slowly come back to enthusiastic gauge;

Enthusiastic softness is the inclination to have a passionate response to occasions that probably won't influence others. For example, on the slight off chance that you are a delicate individual, it probably won't take a lot to make you cry while viewing a sad film or even a program on TV. Or then again, the smallest articulation of inconvenience from somebody near you may cause you to feel like you're being cut in the gut. But, fundamentally, if you are sincerely delicate, you are likely going to respond to most things going on around you, including moderately little things that less touchy individuals probably won't notice.

Passion

Being a sincerely receptive individual implies that, when you respond inwardly, you respond unequivocally, maybe more emphatically than others do. Essentially, you most likely have entirely extraordinary feelings. In this way, in addition to the fact that you have passionate responses to numerous things going on around you, your answers are additionally most likely excellent. Have individuals at any point disclosed to you that you're truly extraordinary? Assuming this is the case, they could be stating that you're genuinely responsive.

Emotional baseline

Slow come back to an emotional baseline implies that once you feel a feeling (for example, outrage), it sets aside an extended effort to leave. For instance, if you had a contention with your supervisor not long before you went home and were feeling angry about it, you would, in all likelihood, despite everything, be feeling angry when you showed up home and welcomed your partner. At that point, if your partner said something that makes you angry, you would be substantially more prone to respond with outrage or to bother because you were already feeling angry with your supervisor.

Escaping your environment

As indicated by the bio-social hypothesis, individuals with BPD are sincerely helpless. However, they additionally experience childhood in conditions where they never figure out how to manage their feelings. Recollect that in a negative situation, individuals don't assist you with figuring out how to manage your feelings. Instead, they may disclose to you that you're off-base for feeling your emotions, or they may rebuff or overlook you when you get enthusiastic.

Individuals don't generally express these things in words; once in a while, their activities convey refutation. For example, envision that you are on the train, and an exceptionally overwhelming individual strides on your foot and remains there; you state, "That truly hurts," and he says, "Indeed, I can see that," however he doesn't move his foot. This is the thing that occasionally occurs in the nullifying condition. Someone accomplishes something that upsets you, you say something regarding it, and the individual continues doing it. For the most part, these are instances of individuals in nature not paying attention to your feelings. Likewise, as previously stated, just experiencing childhood in a family where everybody appears to be unique concerning you can be difficult.

Regardless of whether nobody is letting you know there is some problem with you, you may think there is a significant issue with you—like you are the "odd one." It tends to be highly unbearable to believe that you are extraordinary or softer than others or make some more complicated memories adapting to your feelings. Individuals with BPD regularly have narratives of misuse— physical, emotional, and sexual.

As per the bio-social hypothesis, individuals with BPD have had vast numbers of these encounters growing up. If you have BPD, you may have additionally had the experience of individuals overlooking you, blowing up with you, expelling you, or dismissing you when you got highly enthusiastic. Subsequently, you may have begun to fear your feelings.

Remember, however, that the mix of feeling helplessness and natural refutation is the thing that prompts BPD. Numerous individuals are sincerely powerless. However, they never develop BPD. Thus, numerous individuals have distressing, discrediting, or even harsh childhoods and never produce BPD. It takes two people to dance. It is imperative to take note of that, right now, the factor is to be faulted. There is nothing amiss with being an enthusiastic individual. There are numerous focal points to being progressively passionate.

Now and again, enthusiastic individuals are the most fascinating, magnetic individuals in the room.

They are enthusiastic about existence, profoundly sympathize with others' issues, and are regularly compassionate and delicate. Thus, out of no deficiency of their own, less passionate people may not know precisely how to manage an enthusiastic individual, particularly a passionate youngster.

The kid gets exceptionally enthusiastic, and the parent or parental figures don't have the slightest idea how to manage it. Thus, the parental figures may advise the kid to "quit being so passionate"— not because they need to damage or upset the kid, just because they don't have the slightest idea what to do or how to support the kid.

Right now you're much more enthusiastic than you previously were. What's more important is that your parents currently have even less thought regarding what to do, and they may begin feeling crazy themselves, or even resentful or angry. Consequently, as indicated by the bio-social hypothesis, the two variables are significant, enhancing the other. After some time, as this happens over and over, sincerely powerless individuals may begin to have a great deal of trouble dealing with their feelings, and they may get terrified of their emotions, and invest a ton of energy attempting to stay away from them.

Numerous individuals with BPD state that they do things such as self-damage and suicide endeavors to get away from their feelings. Medication use, voraciously consuming food, and other dangerous practices are likewise utilized for that equivalent reason. Individuals with BPD frequently do these things to feel better for the time being. However, these practices develop an entire group of side issues in the long term.

Approval in DBT
To assist patients with feeling progressively comprehended, DBT utilizes approval. The approval includes checking that individuals are thinking what they are thinking and feeling what they are feeling, just as communicating certified intrigue and comprehension. DBT specialists consistently search for chances to approve their patients'

encounters—to share authentic enthusiasm, understanding, and compassion to their customers.

Acknowledgment in DBT

Through DBT, advisors assist customers with tolerating themselves, the world, their feelings and thoughts, and others by showing abilities, for example, care and procedures for accepting reality for what it is. Tolerating isn't equivalent to favoring, acknowledging, preferring, or craving, and it unquestionably doesn't mean surrendering or giving up. Instead, tolerating is relinquishing the battle to change something and permitting it to be what it is. For instance, when you're genuinely vexed, you might need to change how you feel. That is reasonable.

The issue is that, occasionally, regardless of how hard we attempt, we essentially can't change how we feel. In these situations, trying to change your feelings will make you increasingly upset. Similar procedures work when we are experiencing difficulty tolerating some part of our past. No matter how hard we try, we can't change our history. We can't change the fact that we've done things that make us suffer, that horrible thing that has happened, or that individuals near us have left us. The more we battle to change these things, the more upsetting they become.

Along these lines, tolerating is tied in with dropping the battle to change and simply permitting things to be as they seem to be—in any event until further notice. Acknowledgment doesn't imply that you can't change something that really can be changed. Even though you can't change your history or how you get treated, you can discover approaches to deal with yourself when you get furious and work to take care of individual issues in your relationships and your life.

Problem solving and DBT

DBT is additionally a critical thinking treatment that includes pushing patients to change in manners that are troublesome. DBT is functional and frequently centers on taking care of issues throughout your life. If you are self-destructive and have BPD, at that point, unmistakably something needs to change in your life. Having an advisor who doesn't assist you with changing anything resembles the absurdity. As discussed in the following pages, acknowledgment with no change isn't probably helpful, and change with no acknowledgment doesn't work well indeed, either.

The meaning behind the word "dialectical"

The word dialectical is given the audience's focal point in DBT due to the accentuation on adjusting acknowledgment and change in treatment. An argument is a pressure between perfect inverses—among tremendous and awful, good and bad, or what you want to do (sit on a seashore and drink margaritas, for instance) and what you need to do (go to work). It can be the strain between the need to acknowledge things as they are and the need to change you completely.

Rationalistic hypothesis in DBT centers on how these total inverses meet up and structure something increasingly more complete. For instance, vast numbers of us battle to adjust our job needs with the needs of our family life. We need to invest more energy with our accomplices and our youngsters. Yet, we also feel forced to work extended periods and invest less time with our families to accomplish our goals. Suppose we somehow happened to go totally to the side of our vocations and support the entirety of our energy grinding away. In that case, we may exceed expectations in our career, yet our family life would be wrecked.

Then again, if we somehow happened to invest the entirety of our energy at home with our families, we'd likely be fired. Along these lines, each side is inadequate alone because it doesn't get us what we need throughout everyday life—to be specific, to excel on the two fronts. Logic is how we accomplish these different goals by adjusting contrary energies and uniting them. As another model describes, one of the main goals of a DBT specialist is to adjust acknowledgment of the customer to assist the customer with changing their life.

If your specialist continually pushed you to transform your life, you'd presumably be tired, feel nullified, blow up, and perhaps quit treatment. But, then again, if all your advisor could do was reveal to you how much they understand you, acknowledge you, and know where you are coming from, your treatment most likely wouldn't go anywhere; if you battle with BPD you realize that something needs to change with the goal for you to have an actual existence worth living.

In this way, change alone is deficient because it needs acknowledgment, and acknowledgment is fragmented because it requires change. Therefore, the specialist's goal in DBT is to adjust and unite acknowledgment and change to help the patient.

Chapter 10

Mentalization Based Therapy: a Particular Form of Treatment

In this chapter, we look at another treatment that has been appeared to help individuals with BPD: mentalization-based treatment. MBT hasn't been around as long as DBT has, and it hasn't been concentrated as much either. The primary research on MBT was done in the late 1990s, and, as of this production, a subsequent report was relied upon to be finished in late 2007. As a result, you most likely haven't heard as much about MBT as you have about DBT.

In any case, looking into what has been done on this treatment seems promising. The primary investigation of MBT discovered outcomes that were like outcomes from DBT. These outcomes disclose to us that MBT might be beneficial for individuals with BPD.

MBT

MBT was created by two clinical specialists in England, Dr. Anthony Bateman, and Dr. Dwindle Foray. Also, even though a portion of this treatment is like DBT, it depends on an altogether different thought of what BPD is and how it ought to be dealt with. As you know by now, DBT depends on the bio-social hypothesis. This hypothesis indicates that passionate weakness and issues managing feelings are the absolute most severe issues in BPD.

MBT depends on a different perspective on BPD. Rather than concentrating on issues with feelings, MBT centers on individuals' feelings of what their identity is or their "feeling of self." MBT depends on the possibility that BPD is simply the consequence of a feeble structure or a shaky feeling of self and poor comprehension. Since MBT and DBT depend on such various thoughts of what BPD is and how it develops, it presumably won't shock you that the manners by which these medications look to help individuals are extraordinary.

MBT is a psychoanalytic treatment, not an intellectual, social medicine. This means MBT is, to a greater degree, a "talk treatment." In MBT, the vast majority of your time is spent chatting with your advisor and finding out about yourself and your relationships with others, instead of learning new skills and doing loads of homework assignments, as you would in DBT.

Even though you may leave MBT having gotten some of the equivalent abilities you would get in DBT, you would become familiar with those in a progressively slower manner.

Treatment goals

The second thing that makes MBT not quite the same as DBT is the focal point of the treatment or the treatment goals. As you may recollect from the last part, DBT centers on the most is helping individuals figure out how to manage their feelings in solid manners, rather than doing things that aggravate their issues over the long term (for instance, endeavoring suicide or hurting themselves). Interestingly, the most critical goal in MBT is to build mental structures.

Mental structures give us the capacity to comprehend that our practices and individuals around us emerge from interior mental states, such as musings, emotions, and desires. Essentially, if you have figured out how to do this, you can see that the things you do result from your thoughts, emotions, or desires. These activities are identified with how you feel and the considerations you have.

One of the primary thoughts in MBT is that individuals with BPD make some hard memories seeing how their practices are identified with their psychological states. For instance, individuals with BPD may end up hollering, or drinking, or harming themselves and not know why they began doing those things or what was happening inside them that prompted those practices. If you have BPD, you may feel like your imprudent practices "simply happen." Although it can appear that way, that isn't typically what occurs. Instead, you probably won't know about the sentiments or musings you were having before you began acting incautiously, or you probably won't see the association between your psychological states and your practices.

The fact that you can't see this association doesn't imply that it isn't there; it just means you don't know about it. MBT encourages you to comprehend this association between your psychological states and your practices. Similarly, as it is critical to have the option to see how your practices are identified with your psychological conditions, it is additionally imperative to have the opportunity to see how others' practices come from their psychological states. For instance, suppose that the mother of an adolescent kid hollered at him when she discovered that he had been driving while drunk.

A mental structure would permit the kid to comprehend that his mom was shouting at him since she was frightened and angry. On the slight chance that the kid couldn't understand this, he probably won't see how his mom's shouting was identified with her sentiments and feelings. Mental structures also include the capacity to comprehend that psychological states are identified and separate from conduct simultaneously.

Furthermore, it additionally implies having the option to comprehend what you are thinking, feeling, and needing. Does this last piece sound familiar? That is presumably because understanding what you are feeling and believing is likewise highly significant in DBT as well. This one is where these treatments are very similar. Fundamentally, both of these treatments depend on the possibility that individuals with BPD make some hard memories making sense of what they are feeling and how their emotions and considerations at the time may prompt an assortment of activities.

Dr. Bateman and Dr. Fonagy accept that BPD is brought about by an inability to create mental structures, which prompts issues with the individual's feeling of self (explicitly, a frail self-structure). It's these issues with the self that leads to a significant number of indications of BPD. As per MBT, individuals with BPD are not ready to create mental structures when they are in a condition of enthusiastic excitement or genuinely agitated.

During these occasions, they should turn to different methods for comprehending themselves as well as other people. In particular, since individuals with BPD are not ready to create mental structures during times of extreme pain, they depend on imagination to keep up some feelings of self during unpleasant occasions. Vast numbers of the rash practices that individuals with BPD regularly battle with are believed to be an urgent endeavor to secure oneself and manage the outsider self in some way or another.

For instance, individuals with BPD may get overpowered by the harmful and cruel outsider self-within them. Since having an outsider self is so horrendous, an individual with BPD may hurt themselves with an end goal to obliterate this outsider self (and build up a more grounded or increasingly strong feeling of self). On the other hand, somebody with BPD may attempt to dispose of the outsider self by pushing it outside, into the outer reality (frequently observed as being a piece of another person). Right now, an individual with BPD may lash out at this other individual trying to demolish the outsider self for the last time. As indicated by MBT, this is one of the fundamental reasons individuals with BPD have such stormy connections.

MBT is an extensive treatment that was first evolved as a fractional emergency clinic program. The quantity of hours out of every week spent in therapy in an incomplete clinic program falls somewhere close to inpatient medical clinic projects and standard outpatient treatment.

The MBT incomplete medical clinic program includes six hours of the seven days of organized treatment, including one hour of individual therapy, three-hour-long meetings of group treatment, one hour of treatment, and a network meeting.

Even though the main distributed examinations as of summer 2007 had concentrated on this incomplete clinic program, at press time, Dr. Bateman and Dr. Fonagy were finishing an examination that saw how well MBT fills in as an outpatient treatment program—which would be undeniably progressively functional for by far most of the individuals with BPD.

Chapter 11

Borderline Personality Disorder and Drugs

Numerous individuals with BPD attempt prescriptions—in some cases, a few drugs at the same time. If you are a sincerely exceptional individual, you may have pondered whether a drug could help even out your feelings or cause you to feel quieter or more settled. Or on the other hand, you may have seen TV plugs about drugs that help depression or anxiety and pondered whether these medicines could support you.

This chapter is about prescription drugs for BPD. We talk about various drugs that are once in a while used to treat BPD and a portion of the proof for and against these prescriptions. We talk about a part of the things you should consider on the slight off chance that you are contemplating taking medications, for example, your inclinations concerning drug medicines, drug reactions, and how to get assessed for viable drug treatment.

How medications work

Up until now, we have talked inside and out about mental drugs, which specialists use to assist individuals with improving the nature of their lives by conversing with them, helping them change their practices, musings, and feelings, showing them new adapting aptitudes, or helping them to determine disarranges from quite a while ago. Drug medications vary from mental medicines in that they are proposed to assist individuals with improving the nature of their lives by changing parts of their body or cerebrum science.

Different medications for BPD

For the most part, the most well-known prescriptions utilized for BPD incorporate energizer medicines, state of mind balancing out treatments, and anti-psychotic drugs. This chapter talks about these various sorts of remedies, including how they work and what kinds of symptoms they have. We additionally give you some data about the utilization of these prescriptions for BPD.

Antidepressants

Antidepressants are among the most well-known drugs used to treat BPD. Antidepressants is the name for a massive classification of medicines that are, as anyone might expect, used to treat depression. Generally speaking, individuals use antidepressants to treat BPD because they expect that the downturn side effects and emotional challenges typical among individuals with BPD are the consequence of issues with the synapses serotonin (talked about prior) and norepinephrine. Norepinephrine is a synapse just as a hormone. It is associated with sharpness, fixation, forcefulness, inspiration, and the battle or flight framework.

The general thought is that discouraged individuals need more movement in their norepinephrine or serotonin frameworks; in this manner, most drugs work by expanding action in these zones. However, there are a few unique kinds of drugs. These various kinds of antidepressants work in multiple manners, which we will clarify in the following few pages. For the most part, these medicines fall into four classes: tricycle antidepressants, particular serotonin inhibitors, monoamine oxidase inhibitors, and novel antidepressants.

As you read the following pages, you'll see that we have incorporated a portion of the names of typical antidepressants. The names in brackets toward the finish of each area are the brand names (e.g., Prozac) that you are likely generally acquainted with. One thing that is imperative to recall about these medicines is that in some cases, they require a significant time to kick in and begin assisting with your state of mind. Regularly, it takes two weeks to about a month for antidepressants to start to work.

Tricycle antidepressants (TCAs) work fundamentally by hindering the reuptake of norepinephrine and serotonin. This implies more norepinephrine and serotonin are accessible in the neurotransmitter, and, subsequently, these synapses have a superior possibility of actuating another neuron. A comparative situation occurs with synapses: they get discharged into the neurotransmitter, however sooner or later, they, in some cases, get reclaimed into the neuron that they originated from before they can arrive at the close by neuron and cause it to fire. TCas forestall this procedure of reuptake (being reclaimed into the neuron) for both serotonin and norepinephrine.

Subsequently, more norepinephrine and serotonin are accessible, making these synapses more probable to cause action in specific neurons. Similarly, as with any prescription, it is critical to comprehend what side effects to expect with TCas. A portion of the typical side effects of TCas incorporate the following: dry mouth, weariness, urinary maintenance, tipsiness, obscured vision, hand tremor, obstruction, and nausea. Some normal instances of TCas incorporate amitriptyline (elavil), desipramine (Norpramin), imipramine (Tofranil), nortriptyline (aventyl), and clomipramine (anafranil).

SSRIS

This stands for "Specific serotonin reuptake inhibitors" (SSRIs, for example, Prozac, work in a way that is like that of TCas. Like TCAs, SSRIs forestall the reuptake of serotonin). These drugs keep serotonin from being reclaimed into the neuron it originated from before it gets an opportunity to enact another neuron (called the postsynaptic neuron). The thing that matters is that TCas forestall the reuptake of both serotonin and norepinephrine, though SSRIs prevent the reuptake of serotonin, as it were. Even though the symptoms of SSRIs frequently are very gentle, they are normal. A portion of these reactions incorporates nausea, uneasiness, anxiety, rest aggravation, fretfulness and unsettling, exhaustion, unsteadiness, wooziness, sexual issues (lower sex drive), tremor, dry mouth, perspiring, craziness for individuals who battle with bipolar confusion, weight reduction or weight addition, rashes, and seizures. Some regular instances of SSRIs incorporate fluoxetine (Prozac), sertraline (Zoloft), fluvoxamine (Luvox), citalopram (Celexa), escitalopram (Lexapro), and paroxetine (Paxil).

MAOIs

Monoamine oxidase inhibitors (MAOIs) work such that they are somewhat not the same as TCAs and SSRIs. As we discussed before, the synapses that appear to be generally identified with discouragement are serotonin and norepinephrine. These synapses fall into a classification called monoamine synapses. At the point when monoamine synapses are discharged into the neurotransmitter (the space between two neurons), they have a specific measure of time before synthetic substances in the neurotransmitter separate them, and they are never again ready to tie to and fire the other neuron.

One of the critical synthetic concoctions that separate these synapses is called monoamine oxidase. Along these lines, the MAOIs inhibitor decreases the amount of monoamine oxidase in the neural connection. Accordingly, norepinephrine and serotonin are not separated as fast, and there is a more prominent possibility that these synapses will make it to the next neuron and fire it. Therefore, it is significant for you to think about the symptoms of the MAOIs since they can be more genuine than those of some different antidepressants.

Common symptoms include wooziness, heart changes, stomach steamed, dry mouth, obstruction, and cerebral pains. A portion of the more severe symptoms happens on the slight chance you eat foods or drinks containing amino corrosive called tyramine. Eating such foods and beverages can prompt an extreme hypertensive emergency (where your circulatory strain rises rapidly, and you may encounter the following manifestations: a throbbing migraine, heart palpitations, neck irritation, pallor, chills, nausea, heaving, fretfulness, chest torment, fever, and at times, stroke, unconsciousness, or even death).

You must follow your doctor's dietary proposals if you are taking an MAOI. You'll have to stay away from specific foods and drinks. For example, brew, beer, particular kinds of wine, banana, beans, certain types of cheese, certain meats, particular sorts of fish (particularly smoked fish), ginseng, protein supplements, sauerkraut, certain soups, yeast, and shrimp glue, among different food sources and drinks. A few instances of regular MAOIs incorporate phenelzine (Nardil), tranylcypromine (Parnate), isocarboxazid (Marplan), and selegiline (Eldepryl).

Chapter 12

Dealing with Suicidal Thoughts

If you've followed us this far in the book, you've presumably been thinking about what you can do to manage your issues. We've discussed what BPD is about, the kinds of problems that accompany BPD, how to get treatment, and what sorts of medications are out there. Regardless of whether you want to get treatment soon, it is significant for you to think about the things that you can do to assist yourself with dealing with your feelings, manage worry in your life, and adapt to a portion of the BPD-related issues. We incorporated this part here because, to be completely forthright, if you slaughter yourself, the remainder of these abilities won't work! The most important thing you can do to assist yourself with adapting to your issues is to remain alive.

If you end up contemplating suicide, you might be in a ton of agony a great deal of the time. You may be feeling that taking your life would give an exit from that torment. If this point of view sounds recognizable to you, we should accept that, taking everything into account, you would prefer to remain alive and figure out how to have a less complicated life than end up dead. Remember this as we talk about these abilities. Likewise, remember that pondering suicide and endeavoring suicide can make your life progressively agonizing and increasingly troublesome. In this way, the goal here is to assist you with figuring out how to manage self-destructive considerations (and not follow up on them) when they come up.

The most important tip we can give you is pretty simple: call your doctor as soon as you see these thoughts arising.

What to do if you are feeling suicidal

If you consider on a regular basis, it might be difficult for you to free yourself from these thoughts. It could be possible that your brain becomes used to considering suicide at a point of no return. You may think that it is alleviating to consider suicide, as you might consider it as having a tool that you can utilize if things get tough or if you lose trust. For specific individuals, pondering suicide can become similar to a habit—something awful occurs, and there you have your wrong thought. It tends to be exceptionally hard to change a pattern like this.

Once in a while, the thoughts can come too rapidly for you to have the option to stop them. Therefore, don't expect that you will never again consider suicide. Instead, what may happen is that you will figure out how not to follow up on your thoughts, and you will feel as though you have more opportunity to decide what you do. Beneath, we depict the means you can take on the slight chance of having self-destructive thoughts and thinking about executing yourself.

When you are contemplating suicide, one of the absolute first things you ought to do is escape from deadly treats—anything that you could use to end yourself. Individuals who consider suicide a possibility, as a rule, have to get away from what they would use to execute themselves. If you realize what you would do, at that point, make sure to take yourself away from those deadly methods right away. The idea here is that you are far less inclined to endeavor suicide on the slight off chance that you don't approach the apparatuses or strategies you would use to carry out the responsibility. The following are a few different ways to keep yourself out of dangerous actions.

- If you feel the desire to overdose on your drugs, at that point leave your home and get away from your prescriptions, flush them down the toilet, give them to another person for supervision until the emergency has passed, or lock them up somewhere it would be difficult for you to get them.
- If you feel the desire to hurt yourself with a blade or other sharp items, get these things out of your home, or get yourself away from them.
- Don't let yourself purchase things that you would use to hurt yourself. Try not to let yourself "inadvertently" drive past the store where you could buy highly sharp edges or drugs.
- Don't "inadvertently" end up at your street pharmacist's home where you could purchase drugs for an overdose.

Consider what you want from life
When you have musings about suicide, we recommend that you first consider what you truly need.

The vast majority of people with BPD state that they endeavor suicide to get away from their feelings, or so others would be in an ideal situation. You may be thinking something very similar—that if you murder yourself, you will feel better, you won't need to manage your issues any longer, or you may make it so others wouldn't need to manage you or stress over you any longer. Yet, imagine a scenario where you could take care of those issues and not end up dead.

Consider the possibility of some method for feeling increasingly more calm or content, feeling more in charge of your life, and taking care of your issues. If you notice that you're considering suicide, make sense of what it is you truly need. Then, start by taking the following steps.

- Think, "Goodness, an idea about suicide. This must imply that there's an issue."

- Figure out what the issue is. The problem could be anything. It may be the case that something challenging has simply transpired (for instance, a partner has said a final goodbye to you), and you feel awful and don't know what to do. Or on the other hand, it may be the case that you have felt discouraged for quite a while and can't perceive any exit from it. The significant thing here is to make yourself consider the issue that could be causing these self-destructive musings.

- Figure out what you need. As we have stated before, a great deal of the time, you may very well need your concern to leave, or you should feel progressively content or quiet. Along these lines, instead, state to yourself, "I would prefer not to be dead. I need to do something."

- The next step is to make sense of what you can do to get what you need without executing yourself. If you can't think of something all alone, search for other adapting abilities that may help, call a companion or somebody who can offer you excellent guidance, or talk with your advisor if you have one.

- Remember that murdering yourself is a definitive answer to a transitory issue. Life shocks every one of us from time to time. Imagine a scenario where the response to your concern is simply around the corner, and you never arrive there because you murdered yourself.

At the point when we see individuals who are having self-destructive considerations, frequently the primary thing we ask them is, "Would you like to be dead, or would you like to get away from the torment that you feel in the present moment?" every individual we have suggested this conversation to have stated, "I want to be free from anxiety." Nobody has said, "I want to be dead." Our patients disclose to us that they don't consider suicide because they will likely be dead. Instead, they essentially can't think of another approach to feel good or tackle their issues. They believe suicide to be the solution instead of the problem.

There are numerous different arrangements and approaches to solve the problem. You need to discover them. Furthermore, for that, you may require some assistance— from an advisor, a companion, a relative, a colleague, or maybe a self-improvement guide.

Change the situation

You would be astounded at what a difference simply escaping the environment you are in and into a better place can make. So if you are at home considering suicide, forget about it and head off to someplace, ideally somewhere with others around. In any case, here's the significant thing: don't invest energy pondering heading off to someplace—do what needs to be done.

When you think you have to leave your home (or any place you are right now), choose a safe place and get out now —before you persuade yourself not to do it! Then, at the point when you get to the safe zone, focus on what's happening around you, rather than being latched onto your subconscious mind the entire time.

So focus on the entirety of the sights, sounds, smells, and tastes of everything around you. This will permit you to encounter the world from an alternate point of view. The following is a list of some places you should seriously consider going to when you are feeling self-destructive and need to change your condition immediately.

Where to go when you need to go out
- a shopping center
- a coffeehouse
- a café
- a busy park
- a public place
- a neighbor's home
- a relative's home

Think about positive life experiences

Explanations behind Living/Reasons Not to Commit Suicide:

- Think that you will, at last, have the option to improve your life and take care of your issues in different manners.
- Think that you could hurt your family by murdering yourself
- Think that you would hurt your kids, partner, companions, pets, or others whom you care about if you murdered yourself

It tends to be extremely useful to consider your reasons for not executing yourself. First, glance through this list and check whether any of these reasons are imperative to you. At that point, think of your rundown of reasons. For example, consider how executing yourself will influence the individuals you care about, or consider how murdering yourself may make it hard for your youngsters, family, or pet. Finally, envision the expression on your kid's face if they discover that you executed yourself.

Consider why it bodes well to have trust later on and empower yourself: disclose to yourself that you can go through this and that you will make things change. Focus on the purposes behind living that are critical to you and truly interface with your explanations behind remaining alive.

Frequently, we have discovered that, even in the center of the stormiest emergency, only an idea about a kid or a pet, or only a positive thought, is sufficient to help prevent somebody from endeavoring suicide.

All the more explicitly, self-destructive individuals appear to be more averse to believing that something constructive will occur later than no self-destructive individuals are. They are additionally less ready to think of reasons why adverse occasions won't happen later on. At the point when you are buried in solid, negative feelings, it tends to be unimaginably hard to reason, and miserable reasoning may rule your brain.

Presently, it is likely not simple for you to think positive thoughts on those occasions. When you are in an emergency, the ideal recommended approach to manage miserable believing is to make a move at this moment and abstain from acting sad. When you are thinking sad thoughts, the best actions to make are the ones that reveal to you that things can change.

In Dr. Marsha Lineman's persuasive conduct treatment (PBT), one of the significant techniques used to assist individuals with dealing with their feelings is classified as "inverse activity." This includes acting in a way that is something contrary to what you want to do. In this way, if you are furious and want to scream at somebody, the contrary activity is to be thoughtful to the individual. On the slight chance that you are apprehensive and want to get away from the circumstance, the contrary action is to remain in the present moment.

If you believe that things are bad, at that point, try to do something that you would if you thought everything was fine.

Consider what you would do if you felt cheerful that things could show signs of improvement. At that point, make a move promptly to improve things. You will be unable to take care of your life issues at present. However, you can presumably plan something to cause yourself to feel better, make a slight move to tackle your concern, or work on tolerating what's going on in your life.

Along these lines, when you have sad thoughts, please call a friend, converse with your specialist—do anything you can do to get a thought of the initial step to take. Stepping toward improving things can improve your standpoint and give you trust that things can change. Try not to make a little stride, instead invest the entire energy latched onto your subconscious mind considering how horrendous or sad things are or the amount you'd prefer to murder yourself. Keep your eyes and your brain open to what's going on around you at present, and focus on the little, however significant, advances that you are making.

Allow your thoughts to come and go without holding them in your mind

Another skill that can be exceptionally useful includes letting your self-destructive thoughts travel every which way. The way you're considering suicide doesn't imply that you need to follow up on these thoughts. They are simply thoughts—the movement of your psyche. We as a whole have thoughts that we could never follow up on. For example, you may feel angry with your boss and consider screaming at them or tossing things. However, you don't follow up on these things. We may have had the idea that we'd preferably be eating pizza or sitting on the seashore over composing this book, however on the slight off chance that we had followed up on those thoughts, you wouldn't read this at present. Thoughts are simply thoughts.

From time to time, they can be highly persuading. They sound and feel genuine, and it might appear as though slaughtering yourself is the solution. On the other hand, you have the opportunity to allow your thoughts to travel every which way, and you don't need to follow up on them. The following is one exercise that you can use to rehearse this system:

Imagine that you are lying in an enormous green field and gazing toward the sky. It's a quiet day, warm and radiant, with a slight breeze. In the sky, you see some enormous, surging white mists passing by. Envision that your thoughts are composed on each cloud, and watch the steam as they drift by. Let them go. Try not to follow anyone's shadow (or thought). Let them go.

As we have stated before, numerous individuals with BPD endeavor suicide since they plan to get away from their feelings or the hopelessness of their lives. However, keep in mind that we don't know whether suicide attempts to assist individuals with getting away from their feelings. Furthermore, to have the existence that you need, you need to remain alive. Along these lines, if you're looking for an approach to feel better, at that point, we propose that you use abilities that work. We talk about a portion of these skills in the following chapter.

Chapter 13

Coping with Your Emotions

In this chapter, we will talk about some supportive things you can do to deal with your feelings and get yourself through troublesome occasions.

Utilize these abilities right now to help yourself adapt as you attempt to locate the correct treatment for you, as you are waiting for your treatment to start, or to assist yourself with adjusting to your feelings in any event when you are getting help. Unfortunately, although you can support yourself, there is no proof that self-improvement alone is sufficient to treat BPD.

As you have most likely understood at this point, vast numbers of the issues that individuals with BPD face have to do with feelings. Being an incredibly enthusiastic individual isn't the issue. The problem is the way in which a few people with BPD adapt to their senses. If you have BPD, you may end up doing things imprudently, hurting yourself, or staying away from your feelings no matter what when you feel upset. In any case, as we've previously stated, although doing these things may work for the time being, they will, in general, reason entirely significant issues in the long haul. Hurting yourself may cause you to feel better for some time. However, it can likewise break your dignity, lead to perpetual scars, and keep you attached to harming yourself as an approach to adapt to life.

Evading your feelings may work for the time being. Yet, you will presumably wind up feeling far worse in the long haul if you generally maintain a strategic distance from your feelings.

Accept your emotions without fighting them

One of the easiest practices to manage feelings is to work on tolerating the emotions you are encountering, accepting the troublesome circumstance you are in, or handling the upsetting things that have happened to you. We called it "practice" because tolerating your feelings is genuinely something that you progress in the direction of, as opposed to something that you accomplish. Tolerating isn't care for finishing an end-of-the-year test and being finished with a course; it's increasingly similar to cleaning your home. In contrast to cleaning your home, in any case, you can't get another person to acknowledge your feelings for you.

Distract yourself from your thoughts

At times, the ideal approach to manage your feelings when you are genuinely disturbed is to concentrate on something different. Distraction is discovering another thing to focus on that gets your psyche off of whatever is alarming you. This can be a great tool to overcome the most difficult moments.